ESSENTIAL GUIDE

DRUGS &
FIRST AID

ESSENTIAL GUIDE

DRUGS &
FIRST AID

This edition first published in 1995

© Bloomsbury Publishing Plc

A copy of the CIP entry for this book is available from the British Library

ISBN 1 8598 0011 4

10 9 8 7 6 5 4 3 2 1

Cover design by Planet X
Edited, designed and typeset by Book Creation Services, London
Printed in Britain by HarperCollins Manufacturing, Glasgow

CONTENTS

All about drugs

PAGE 7

A to Z of drugs and drug actions

PAGE 75

First aid

PAGE 505

All about drugs

Introduction to the therapeutic and harmful effects of drugs

The information in this chapter is not to be considered as a guide to self-medication, nor to be used as a substitute for skilled professional prescribing. Many more factors are involved in the medical treatment of disease than can be dealt with here. But many people for whom medication is prescribed like to take an informed interest in the effects – intended and otherwise – of the drugs they are taking.

CONTENTS

What is a drug?   10

Administering drugs   14

Risk versus benefit   20

Over-the-counter drugs   28

A selection of proprietary remedies   30

Drug abuse   47

WHAT IS A DRUG?

The term 'drug', as used in medicine, covers every substance taken into the body, by any route, to exert some desired effect. Any chemical compound used to treat or prevent disease, relieve symptoms or even to help in the diagnosis of disease, is a drug. Today, there remain almost no diseases for which there is no drug treatment, either to cure or relieve symptoms.

Drugs are used to relieve pain or discomfort and to regularize and control abnormal conditions of mind and body. Some drugs act on cells within the body, often by influencing the many receptors on the cell membranes or within the cells. Others act on the various agencies which can harm the body, such as bacteria, viruses, fungi and other parasites of many kinds. Drugs are commonly used to suppress or modify normal physiological action in the body states, as in the use of oral contraceptives.

The most powerful, and hence potentially dangerous, drugs can be obtained only on a doctor's prescription. Some are subject to strict regulations governing storage, recording of stocks held, methods of prescription, and so on. Nonprescription, or 'over-the-counter' drugs can be bought, without restriction, in a pharmacist's shop. They are, in general, reasonably safe even if the recommended dose is somewhat exceeded, but it should be remembered that any drug, however seemingly innocuous, can be dangerous if taken in large excess.

To try to help to reduce the horrendous drug bill of the National Health Service in the UK, government has progressively increased the number of drugs, formerly prescription-only, that can be bought over-the-counter. There are dangers in this as these drugs were not initially restricted without good reason. Advice on such drugs can be obtained from pharmacists.

Drug names

A generic drug is the 'official', approved, nonproprietary, and usually cheaper form of a single substance. The generic name is nearly always different from the name under which the drug is marketed (the trade or brand name), and there is often a range of different proprietary names –

and prices – for the identical generic drug.

Thus, 'paracetamol' is the generic name of the common pain-killing (analgesic) drug Panadol, also known by many other names including Calpol, Pamol, Panasorb and Salzone. To make matters worse, the generic name of a drug is seldom a true chemical name. Acetaminophen, which is also paracetamol, sounds like a chemical name, but 4'-Hydroxyacetanilide is the real chemical name of

---

Generic drugs

A generic drug – is a drug sold under the official medical name of the basic active substance. The generic name is chosen by the Nomenclature Committee of the British Pharmacopoeia Commission and is used in publications such a the National Formulary. Doctors are encouraged to prescribe generic drugs as these are generally cheaper than the same drug under a trade name.

paracetamol. Some of the brand names given in this book are used only in the USA and Australia; most are British.

Many proprietary preparations contain mixtures or combinations of generic drugs. Paracetamol is one of the main agents in Cafadol, Carisoma Co, Cosalgesic, Delimon, Distalgesic, Femerital, Fortagesic, Lobak, Medocodene, Myolgin, Neurodyne, Norgesic, Paedo-sed, Paracodol, Panadeine, Parahypon, Parake, Paralgin, Paramol-118, Para-selzer, Parazolidin, Pardale, Paxidal, Pharmidone, Propain, Safapryn, Solpadeine, Syndol, Tandalgesic, Unigesic, Veganin and Zactipar.

These pain-killing preparations also include drugs such as aspirin, caffeine, codeine and phenylbutazone. Official publications, such as the British National Formulary express disapproval of these compound preparations, as they tend unnecessarily to increase the cost of treatment and may make it more difficult for doctors dealing with cases of overdosage.

All drugs of medical value are available in the generic form and a few doctors prescribe generic drugs only.

ADMINISTERING DRUGS

Drugs can be given in a surprising number of different ways.

Skin

Drugs can be applied to the skin in the form of ointments, creams, lotions, powders or solutions. Although, in general, such drugs act only on the skin and are not absorbed in sufficient quantity to have an effect on the rest of the body, in some cases significant absorption occurs.

Powdered drugs applied to large raw areas or to ulcers can be dangerously absorbed. Skin patches, from which drugs are slowly absorbed, have become popular for certain drugs. This route is used for hormone replacement therapy, for contraception and for an increasing number of other purposes.

Injections

Drugs may be given by injection into the skin, using a very fine needle (an intradermal injection), just under the skin (a subcutaneous injection), deeply into a muscle (an intramuscular injection) or into the blood flowing in a vein (an intravenous injection). Drugs given by injection usually act more quickly than drugs taken by mouth. Drugs given intravenously may act within seconds.

Injection may be necessary for a number of reasons. A drug may be so urgently required that the oral route would take too long. Many drugs, if taken by mouth, would be destroyed by the stomach acid or the digestive enzymes.

Some drugs are so damaging to tissues that the only way they can safely be given is by slow intravenous injection so that they are rapidly diluted by, and carried away in, the passing blood. Deep intramuscular injections allow larger volumes to be given than can comfortably be accommodated under the skin.

This allows a longer period of action. An even longer-acting effect can be achieved by formulating drugs in a vehicle – such as an oil or a wax – from which absorption is particularly slow. These are called depot injections.

Many different drugs and hormones may be given in depot form. They include antibiotic drugs, corticosteroid drugs, antipsychotic drugs, sex hormones and contraceptive drugs. Injections are not routinely given into arteries.

Sometimes drugs are given in the form of implants – small tablets or other formulations which are buried under the skin through a tiny incision closed with one or two small stitches.

Long-acting contraceptives are often given in this form. Injections are occasionally given into the bone marrow, into the cerebro-spinal fluid surrounding the spinal cord, or into the abdominal cavity.

Drugs by mouth

Drugs to be taken by mouth are formulated in various ways. These include:

◆ coated or uncoated tablets;
◆ cylindrical, two-piece capsules which are slid open to insert the drug in powder or granuleform;
◆ sealed gelatin ovoids containing a liquid;
◆ soft rolled pills;
◆ flat cachets of rice-paper or other material.

Tablets come in all sizes and shapes, are often colour-coded, and may have manufacturer's identifying particulars impressed or printed on them. Capsules are also often colour-coded. Sometimes the two halves of capsules are differently coloured. Within capsules, individual granules may be of one or more colours.

Because of the permutations of size, shape, colour and form, it is often possible for an expert to identify a drug from the appearance of the formulation. Tablet- and capsule-identification tables are available to assist doctors dealing with poisoning cases.

Oral drugs are not necessarily intended to be swallowed. Some drugs are actually absorbed more rapidly if kept in the mouth. Nitroglycerine for angina, for instance, works more quickly if the tablet is put under the tongue than if it is swallowed.

Some drugs, such as aspirin and alcohol, are absorbed from the stomach, but most pass on to the small intestine, which is the normal absorption zone for food.

Some drugs are less well absorbed if mixed with food and are prescribed to be taken 'on an empty stomach'. Others are irritating to the intestinal tract and are best taken immediately

17

after a meal. In general, this is not a very important matter.

Drugs likely to cause severe stomach irritation are often given in a capsule made of a material which will not dissolve until it reaches the small intestine. These are called 'enteric-coated' capsules. A wide range of 'slow-release' formulations is available, usually in capsule form containing layers of the drug, or tiny spherules, each coated with a protective covering.

Drugs by inhalation

Many drugs may be rapidly absorbed into the circulation, or have local effect, if inhaled in aerosol or fine powder form. Nicotine from cigarette smoke, for instance, reaches the brain within a few seconds of inhalation. Inhalation from inhalers is an important route of access for drugs in such conditions as asthma, and allows drugs to reach the desired areas in high concentration, while minimizing general effects.

Other routes

Drugs may gain access to the circulation through any absorbent surface. Some drugs are usefully administered, in the form of rectal suppositories, from which absorption is effective. These bullet-shaped medications are moulded from a substance such as cocoa butter, with which the drug is mixed, and which melts at body temperature. They are easily passed in through the anus. Similar vaginal pessaries may be administered usually for local action against vaginal infections.

Drugs may also be absorbed from the nose lining, from the conjunctiva of the eyes, or from the inside of the bladder or urine tube (urethra). These routes, however, are not generally employed if full absorption is desired, but are normally used so that the drug can act locally.

RISK VERSUS BENEFIT

Drugs with powerful and valuable actions are seldom if ever free from risk. Doctors are always aware of this and do not prescribe unless the benefit is likely to outweigh the risk. In most cases, the risks are small and the doctor is in no doubt, but sometimes, especially in cases of severe illness, the risk may be only a little less than the risk of leaving the disease untreated. This can make for difficult decisions.

Anticancer drugs, for instance, are always poisonous (toxic) and usually have severe and often unpleasant side-effects. This is because they are intended to destroy cells and their damaging effect on cancer cells may not be very much greater than on normal cells. No effective anticancer drug can avoid damaging healthy cells to some extent. In such a case, however, even a small margin of benefit over risk (the therapeutic ratio) may be gladly accepted.

Doctors are often criticized for the overuse of powerful drugs, such as antibiotics, and it is probably true that the best doctors prescribe these and other drugs less often than some of their colleagues. But doctors are extremely busy people and very often they find they have insufficient time to carry out a full examination and a range of tests. So they may be driven by discretion to prescribe 'just in case'. Family doctors do not have immediate access to the facilities enjoyed by hospital doctors.

Drug side-effects

A side effect is any action not intended, and there are many of these. Different drugs may cause different side-effects and these include nausea, vomiting, loss of appetite, diarrhoea, constipation, drowsiness, tiredness, a dry mouth, blurring of vision, a rapid heartbeat, difficulty in urinating, even impotence. Some may lower the blood pressure and cause fainting. There may be upset of the menstrual cycle.

Drugs acting on the central nervous system, such as sedatives, narcotics and tranquillizers, commonly affect mood, judgement, memory and motivation in an adverse way, and may also disturb bodily coordination.

Drug allergy is not, strictly, a side-effect, but

to those suffering allergic reactions to drugs, the distinction may seem academic. Allergy may manifest itself as a skin rash, itching, the raised, purplish swellings of urticaria, asthma, complete blockage of the airway from swelling of the lining of the voice box, intestinal upset, fainting, shock or collapse. Drug allergy is especially dangerous when the drug concerned is given by injection, and doctors are always wary of this. Usually a very small test dose is given first and then, after an interval, if nothing untoward happens, the full dose.

Allergic reactions do not occur the first time a drug is given, as the sensitivity must be acquired from a previous exposure. But allergy can be acquired from a drug with a completely different name from the drug now being given, but which happens to belong to the same group, or even to be identical. This is one of the many disadvantages of the present chaotic system of naming drugs.

Drug toxicity

Poisoning by drugs is common, usually because of excessive quantities of the drug in the body. This may be because the drug is given in excessive dosage or because, although dosage is normal, the rate of loss of the drug, by breakdown or excretion, is reduced. Kidney disease, for instance, commonly prevents normal excretion.

The liver is especially liable to drug toxicity because it is exposed to high concentrations of most drugs. Hepatitis, even liver atrophy and failure, can be caused by drugs. The kidneys, too, in their attempts to get rid of drugs, may suffer a high concentration and be exposed to toxic levels. In the days of the sulphonamides, these drugs used sometimes to occur in such high concentrations in the urine that they formed damaging crystals within the kidneys or the ureters. Drugs can cause blindness, by retinal or optic nerve toxicity, and deafness, by damage to the sensitive hair cells in the cochlea of the inner ear.

The thalidomide disaster is too well known to require comment, but it has now alerted all concerned to the high sensitivity of the young fetus, especially in the first three months of life, to any possibly damaging agency which can gain access to it. As a result, prescribing to women in early pregnancy is now, rightly, very cautious.

Many drugs are habit-forming and this must be balanced against their advantages. 'Sleeping pills', once widely and freely prescribed, are now used with much greater caution. The same applies to sedative drugs such as the diazepams (e.g., Valium), the barbiturates and opiate drugs such as morphine and the wide range of powerful pain-killers such as methadone.

Accidental or suicidal poisoning from drugs is very common and child-proof packaging methods are now routinely employed. Some drugs commonly used in suicide attempts are being combined with an antidote.

Drug interactions

Regrettably, many people have to take more than one drug at a time, and drugs are very occasionally prescribed without adequate knowledge of what the patient may already be taking. Drug interactions are the effects of such simultaneous dosage, and they may be dangerous. Interaction may increase the toxicity or reduce the effectiveness of the drugs.

The commonest interaction is well known – the additive effect of similar drugs or of drugs having similar actions – and the commonest example is the additive effect of alcohol on any of the sedatives or tranquillizers. This can lead to a dangerous degree of sedation, and may, for instance, make driving hazardous. The law does not excuse a transgressor, and links 'drink' and 'drug' in its proscription.

Sometimes drugs combine to reduce the effect of both. One drug may interfere with the absorption of another. Drugs are commonly bound to, and carried by, proteins in the blood. One drug can sometimes displace another from its bound form, releasing it for greater activity.

Much of what happens in cells is controlled by thousands of different enzymes. Drugs can interfere with enzyme action, either enhancing or interfering with it. The action of liver enzymes can be increased by barbiturates. Drugs are often broken down by enzymes, so that the duration of their action is limited. Some other drugs, by interfering with the action of these breaking-down enzymes, allow the first drug to act for much longer than normal. Some drugs prevent the action of others by blocking the receptor sites on cell membranes where drugs act.

Drugs and the elderly

In general, elderly people take more drugs, and have more trouble from prescribed drugs, than younger people. Because old age commonly brings multiple disorders, there is a natural tendency to multiple prescribing – tablets for the heart, for the blood pressure, for arthritic pain, for insomnia, for swelling (oedema) of the ankles and fluid in the lungs, and for urinary infections. Many old people are taking more than four separate remedies, some as many as ten.

Elderly people tend to have faith in medicines and will often buy additional remedies from a chemist's or even take medicines recommended and given them by their friends, from a well-stocked bathroom cabinet. Like conventional drugs, herbal remedies contain active and potentially harmful ingredients and overuse of these can add to the problem. They may even interact with prescribed medication.

Doctors concerned about this problem have made searching investigations and these have brought to light some horrifying facts – old people being seriously overdosed, suffering severe drug interactions (see above), taking medicines whose actions cancel one another out, and so on.

Often more than one doctor is involved and sometimes each is unaware of what the other has been prescribing. It has been found that in rare cases some confusional states, diagnosed as senile dementia or Alzheimer's disease, have been due to overtreatment with tranquillizers.

It is wise for people in this situation, who are about to visit a doctor, to write down the name of everything they are taking and how many per day. If possible, the reason for the medication should also be recorded. Non-prescription drugs being taken should be included, as should complementary remedies.

OVER-THE-COUNTER DRUGS

These are drugs that you can buy without prescription. This is not to imply that such drugs are harmless; many of these OTC preparations contain powerful drugs, and they should all be used responsibly and in the exact dosage recommended. Government decisions to save money in this way have not been uniformly approved by doctors. To quote from a Lancet leading article in June, 1994: 'The unthinkable is happening at the pharmacy counter. Drugs that no one would have dreamed would take the route can be bought over-the-counter (OTC), and more will follow...'

In Britain, the following are some of the potent drugs that can now be bought over-the-counter:

◆ various non-sedating antihistamine drugs;
◆ some steroid drugs for hay fever;

- ◆ nicotine patches;
- ◆ acyclovir cream for herpes simplex;
- ◆ imidazole antifungal drugs;
- ◆ hydrocortisone cream;
- ◆ sodium cromoglycate eyedrops;
- ◆ H2 receptor antagonists;
- ◆ various non-steroidal anti-inflammatory drugs (NSAIDs).

It seems likely that various antibiotics for local use, chloromycetin (chloramphenicol) eye drops and some anti-emetic drugs will also soon be available OTC.

There is a strong lobby to make oral contraceptives available over-the-counter. These recently released drugs are obtainable only from a registered pharmacy where advice can be obtained from the pharmacist. Doctors anticipate that pharmacists will spend more time talking to customers than before.

Doubts have been expressed about the safety of some of these changes, mainly on the grounds that patients may be denied the advice normally given by a doctor when such drugs are prescribed.

Concern has also been voiced over the risk of

adverse interactions of these drugs with prescribed drugs. Some doctors are worried that symptoms of a more serious disorder may be concealed by the use of such drugs. Others, however, view the change favourably.

A great many drugs have long been available over-the-counter in the form of proprietary medicines, available anywhere. The following list is a selection of these remedies, taken from the monthly price list of the *Chemist and Druggist* journal.

They are listed under brand names and show the active ingredients, the action of which can be found in the *A to Z of Drugs and Drug Actions*. It is interesting to note how often the same drugs appear in this list.

A selection of proprietary remedies

Actifed Compound Linctus

triprolidine, pseudoephedrine, dextromethorphan

Actifed Expectorant

triprolidine, pseudoephedrine, guiaphenesin

Actifed Syrup

triprolidine, pseudoephedrine

Aller-eze
clemastine hydrogen fumarate

Aller-eze Plus
clemastine, phenylproanolamine

Altacite
hydrotalcite

Altacite Plus
hydrotalcite, dimethicone

Aludrox
aluminium hydroxide

Anadin
aspirin, caffeine, quinine

Anadin Extra
aspirin, caffeine, paracetamol

Anadin Ibuprofen
ibuprofen

Andrews Answer
paracetamol, caffeine, sodium bicarbonate, citric
acid

Andrews Liver salts
sodium bicarbonate, citric acid, magnesium sulphate

Asilone
dimethicone, aluminium hydroxide, magnesium oxide

Aspro
aspirin

Aspro Clear
aspirin

Aspro Paraclear
paracetamol

Beechams Capsules
paracetamol, caffeine, phenylephrine

Beecham Coughcaps
dextromethorphan

Beechams Hot Lemon
paracetamol, ascorbic acid, phenylephrine

Beechams Pills
aloin

Beechams Powders
aspirin, caffeine

Beechams Tablets
aspirin

Benylin
diphenhydramine, menthol, dextromethorphan

Benylin with Codeine
diphenhydramine, codeine, sodium citrate,
menthol

Biactol Face Wash
sodium lauryl, ether sulphate, phenoxypropanol

Bisodol Extra
calcium carbonate, light magnesium carbonate,
sodium bicarbonate, dimethicone

Bisodol Powders
sodium bicarbonate, heavy and light magnesium
carbonate

Bisodol Tablets
calcium carbonate, light magnesium carbonate, sodium bicarbonate

Bradosol lozenges
benzalkonium chloride

Bradosol Plus lozenges
domiphen bromide, lignocaine

Brolene Eye Drops
propamidine isethinate, benzalkonium chloride, phenylethanol

Brolene Ointment
dibromopropamidine isethionate

Bronalin (dry cough)
dextromethorphan, pseudoephedrine, alcohol

Bronalin (expectorant)
diphenhydramine, sodium citrate, ammonium chloride

Coldrex
paracetamol, phenylephrine, ascorbic acid

Collis Browne's Mixture
morphine anhydrous, peppermint oil

Collis Browne's Tablets
light kaolin, morphine, heavy calcium carbonate

Cupal Cold Sore Lotion
povidone iodine

Cupal Cold Sore Ointment
diperodone hydrochloride

Cupal Corn Solvent
salicylic acid

Cupal Nail Bite Cream
bitrex, turpentine, menthol, eucalyptus oil,
allantoin, camphor, zinc oxide

Cupal Wart Solvent
concentrated acetic acid

Dettol Cream
chloroxylenol, triclosan, edetic acid

Dettol Liquid
chloroxylenol

Dettol Mouthwash
cetylpyridinium chloride

Dettol Soap
trichlorocarbanilide

De Witt's antacid powders
magnesium trisilicate, light magnesium carbonate, calcium carbonate, sodium bicarbonate, light kaolin, peppermint oil

De Witt's antacid tablets
magnesium trisilicate, magnesium carbonate, calcium carbonate, peppermint oil, lactose

De Witts lozenges
tyrothricin, benzocaine, cetylpyridinium chloride

De Witt's pills
paracetamol, caffeine

Dimotane
brompheniramine maleate

Dimotane Co
brompheniramine maleate, pseudoephedrine, codeine

Dimotane Expectorant
brompheniramine maleate, guiaphenesin, phenylephrine, phenylpropanolamine

Dimotane Plus
brompheniramine maleate, pseudoephedrine

Diocalm
morphine, attapulgite

Diocalm Ultra
loperamide

Diprobase Cream
chlorocresol

Diprobase Ointment
liquid paraffin, white soft paraffin

Disprin
aspirin

Disprin Extra
aspirin, paracetamol

Eludril Mouthwash
chlorhexidine digluconate, chlorbutol
hemihydrate

Eludril Spray
chlorhexidine digluconate, amethocaine

Expulin Cough linctus
pholcodine, pseudoephedrine, chlorpheniramine
maleate

Expulin Linctus
pholcodine

Famel Expectorant
guaiphenesin

Famel Linctus
pholcodine

Fedril Expectorant
diphenhydramine, ammonium chloride, menthol

Fedril Liquid
cetyl pyridinium chloride, ipecacuanha, lemon oil, honey, ammonium chloride, glycerin, citric acid

Fennings Gripe Mixture
sodium bicarbonate, peppermint oil, dill oil, caraway oil

Fennings Lemon Mixture
sodium salicylate

Fennings Little Healers
ipecacuanha

Fennings Powders
paracetamol

Fiery Jack Cream
glycol salicylate, diethylamine salicylate, capsicum oleoresin, methyl nicotinate

Fiery Jack Ointment
capsicum oleoresin

Flurex Capsules
paracetamol, phenylephrine

Flurex Liquid (bedtime)
paracetamol, diphenhydramine, pseudoephedrine

Flurex Liquid (hot lemon)
codeine, diphenhydramine, ephedrine

Flurex Tablets
paracetamol, phenylephrine, caffeine

Franolyn Expectorant
ephedrine, guiaphenesin, theophylline

Franolyn SED
dextromethorphan

Galfer
ferrous fumarate

Galpseud
pseudoephedrine

Gaviscon Sachets
sodium alginate, magnesium alginate, aluminium hydroxide

Gaviscon Tablets
alginic acid, sodium bicarbonate, calcium carbonate

Gelcotar Gel
coal tar, pine tar

Gelcotar Shampoo
coal tar, cade oil

Germolene Cream
chlorhexidine gluconate

Germolene Ointment
lanolin, soft paraffins, liquid paraffin, starch, zinc
oxide, methyl salicylate, octaphonium chloride,
phenol

Germolene Spray
triclosan, dichlorophen

Germoloids
lignocaine, zinc oxide

Hydromol Bath Additive
liquid paraffin, isopropyl myristate

Hydromol Cream
calamine, zinc oxide, zinc carbonate,
hahamelis water

Lana-sting Cream
lignocaine, benzyl alcohol

Lana-sting Spray
benzocaine, benzethonium chloride

Lem-Plus Capsules
paracetamol, caffeine, phenylephrine

Lem-Plus Powders
paracetamol, ascorbic acid

Lemsip
paracetamol, dextromethorphan,
chlorpheniramine, phenylpropanolamine

Mac Extra Lozenges
hexylresorcinol

Mac Lozenges
amylmetacresol, menthol, sucrose, glucose

Mu-Cron Syrup
phenylpropanolamine, ipecacuanha

Mu-Cron Tablets
phenylpropanolamine, paracetamol

Mycil Footspray
tolnaftate

Mycil Ointment
tolnaftate, benzalkonium chloride

Mycil Powder
tolnaftate, chlorhexidine

Mycota Cream
zinc undecanoate, undecanoic acid

Mycota Spray
undecanoic acid, dichlorophen

Oilatum Cream
arachis oil, povidone iodine

Oilatum Emollient
liquid paraffin, acetylated wood alcohols

Oilatum Gel
light liquid paraffin

Phytocil Cream
phenoxypropanol, chlorphenoxyethanol, zinc
undecanoate

Quinoderm Cream
potassium hydroxyquinolone sulphate, benzoyl peroxide

Quinoderm Face Wash
chlorhexidine gluconate, cetrimide, sodium N-lauroyl sacosinate, lauric diethanolamide

Ralgex Cream
methyl nicotinate, capsicin

Raglex Spray
glycol monosalicylate, ethyl salicylate, methyl salicylate, capsicin, menthol

Rennies
calcium carbonate, magnesium carbonate

Rennies Gold
calcium carbonate

Robitussin
dextromethorphan

Robitussin Expectorant
guiaphenesin

Robitussin Plus
guiaphenesin, pseudoephedrine

Savlon Cream
cetrimide, chlorhexidine gluconate

Ster-Zac Liquid
triclosan

Ster-Zac Powder
hexachlorophane

Sudafed Expectorant
guiaphenesin, pseudoephedrine

Sudafed Linctus
dextromethorphan, pseudoephedrine

Throaties Linctus
glycerol, honey, citric acid

Tixylix Cough and Cold Linctus
pseudoephedrine, chlorpheniramine maleate,
pholcodine

Ulcaid Gel
lignocaine, alcohol, cetylpyridinium chloride

Ulcaid Tablets
tyrothricin, benzocaine, cetylpyridinium chloride

Valderma Cream
potassium hydroxyquinolone sulphate, chlorocresol

Valderma Soap
trichlorocarbanilide

Venos (dry cough)
glucose, treacle, aniseed oil, capsicum, camphor

Venos Expectorant
guiaphenesin, glucose, treacle, aniseed oil,
capsicum, camphor

Venos Honey Lemon
lemon juice, honey, glucose

DRUG ABUSE

What is it?

There is some general confusion as to what is meant by the term 'drug', and, in the context of drug abuse, most people think of narcotic drugs such as heroin or stimulating drugs such as cocaine. But such restriction is arbitrary. A drug is any substance, other than a food, which affects the body in any way.

Thus the term includes tobacco (nicotine), alcohol (ethanol) and coffee and tea (caffeine). Most people are habitual drug takers and many of them are addicted to these drugs. This kind of indulgence is not generally regarded as 'abuse'. Most heavy tea drinkers would seriously resent being described as drug abusers. So the mere regular indulgence in a drug can hardly be described as drug abuse.

What is acceptable?

There are many people who, likewise, do not

consider the occasional use of substances like marijuana (cannabis) or cocaine as abuse. In many parts of the world, drugs, such as betel nut, pan or opium are used by many, habitually and in reasonable moderation, and doubtless these people would not consider themselves as abusing a drug. But no one would deny that there are many who do abuse alcohol and tobacco, to the detriment of their health.

And there are millions who, with or without the tacit connivance of doctors, abuse drugs such as valium or librium (benzodiazepines), equanil (meprobamate) and many others.

So the phrase drug abuse is unclear and unsatisfactory. One might consider that abuse exists if the drug harms the body. However, the potent drug more widely used than any other throughout the world – nicotine – appears to be almost harmless to the body.

The fact that people who take nicotine by smoking cigarettes are probably engaging in the most harmful long-term activity available to them is, in this context, neither here nor there. It is the many other substances in the smoke that do the harm, and the smoker is not addicted to these. So the matter is more complicated than it at first appears.

Socially unacceptable drugs

In fact, drug abuse has come to mean the use of any drug which is currently disapproved of by the majority of the members of a society. In an attempt to clarify the concept of drug abuse, the class of drugs used to alter the state of the mind for recreational or pleasure purposes is often divided into 'hard drugs' and 'soft drugs'. The

---

Remember

It is important to appreciate that classification into 'hard' or 'soft' is in no way an indication of relative safety. For it is clear that, at least at the present stage of social development, the abuse of 'soft' drugs, such as alcohol and tobacco kills many times more people than abuse of 'hard' drugs.

distinction is somewhat arbitrary, but hard drugs are those which are liable to cause major emotional and physical dependency and thus an alteration in the social functioning of the user.

This group includes heroin, morphine and pharmacologically similar natural or synthetic substances. The soft drug group includes tranquillizers, sedatives, cannabis, amphetamines, alcohol, hallucinogens and tobacco.

Damaging effects

The term 'drug abuse' might thus be more usefully taken to mean the use of any substance in such quantity or frequency that it leads to physical, mental or social damage to the user or to others. Such damage is not always obvious.

One important element in it, which applies to all drugs and which may be the central reason why drug abuse is undesirable, is this: people who rely on seriously psychoactive drugs deprive themselves, to a greater or lesser degree, of the opportunity to solve their own problems by personal constructive effort.

For such people, it is easier to take a drug than to face up to personal difficulties, analyse them, and plan and execute solutions. It is easier to take a drug than to develop their own capacity for interest, appreciation and enjoyment through the acquisition of knowledge. It is easier to take a drug than to work.

Cocaine and crack

INCIDENCE

The world is experiencing a pandemic of stimulant drug usage. This is the fifth, and largest, epidemic of stimulant abuse – mainly cocaine or amphetamine and its derivatives – and all have run to the same pattern. Initially, the drug is widely claimed to be harmless.

Then, as usage extends more and more widely, clear evidence of the dangers arises and reasonable people are frightened off. Usage then declines. Previous episodes occurred in the 1890s, the 1920s, the early 1950s and the late 1960s. The current flare-up threatens to be different, and not only quantitatively. It is being fuelled by criminal interests, aware of the unlimited profits to be made from an increasingly affluent society.

The age of first use is dropping, as are street prices, and the numbers of people being treated for the medical consequences is rising steeply. Cocaine-related deaths in the United States have risen to around five per 1000.

Crack is a highly purified and powerful form of cocaine, volatile on heating and readily absorbed through the lungs. It acts similarly to amphetamine, causing a 'high' with a short period of intense pleasure. This feeling is strongest on the first use and is never experienced to the same intensity again.

Crack quickly leads to dependence in some users and there is no way of knowing, in advance, who will become addicted and who will not. Some people seem to have little difficulty in keeping usage under control, but about 15 per cent of users go on taking larger and larger doses until they are as dependent as heroin addicts.

Animals given the choice of injecting themselves with cocaine or taking food, prefer the cocaine and continue to inject until they are exhausted or dead. Human cocaine users, of course, have the advantage over the animals of choosing to apply reason.

ADDICTION

The likelihood of severe addiction depends on the way the drug is used. People who are into 'freebasing' (smoking) or 'shooting' (injecting) are more likely to become seriously addicted than those who are only 'snorting' the drug.

The trouble is that habituation and tolerance to the effect may lead snorters to want the extra 'rush' of freebasing, in which 80 per cent of the dose can get to the brain in about ten seconds. As with any other major drug, addiction, quite apart from its medical effects, may lead to serious social and financial consequences.

RISKS

There is now ample medical evidence to show that cocaine is often extremely dangerous to health. The commonest serious physical effects are epileptic-type fits, loss of consciousness – 'tripping out' – unsteadiness, sore throat, running and bleeding nose, sinusitis, pain in the chest, coughing blood, pneumonia, severe itching ('the cocaine bug'), irregularity of the heart, loss of appetite and stomach upset.

Some of the chest and throat problems are probably caused by the high temperature of the inhaled cocaine fumes.

The nose and sinus disorders are due to the constricting effect of cocaine on the blood vessels in the nose linings.

This is followed by rebound swelling, but is sometimes severe enough to destroy part of the partition between the two halves of the nose, leaving a perforation.

Crack, like amphetamine, can lead to a short-lived, acute form of mental illness. This is called a cocaine psychosis. The symptoms include severe depression, agitation, delusions, ideas of persecution, hallucinations, violent behaviour and suicidal intent. People with a cocaine psychosis often have 'lucid intervals' in which they seem normal and will often deny using the drug. Cocaine psychosis usually follows long binges or high doses.

Anyone who thinks cocaine usage safe and amusing, is either ignorant or extremely foolish.

Designer drugs

The lucrative market in 'recreational' drugs has prompted people, unburdened by social conscience, to exploit their chemical and pharmacological expertise for illicit gain. The chemistry of many of the drugs of addiction and stimulation is well known, and it is not very difficult to modify other substances so as to produce seemingly new drugs not covered by existing prohibitive legislation. These 'designer drugs' are often modifications of respectable medical products and are produced in secret laboratories without regard to their obvious dangers or to the possible unknown toxic effects of modified substances. Some may cause sterility. They can often be produced very cheaply and can be sold on the street at lower prices than existing drugs. Their manufacturers and purveyors look for legal protection on the specious basis that they are new.

Legislators recognize that the young, the foolish and the irresponsible, who are the prey of such people, require protection against them. The designer drug movement is already attracting some rigorous attention. Drugs such as the fentanyl analogues (e.g., 'China white') and the amphetamine derivatives (e.g., 'Ecstasy') have already been covered by legislation in the USA.

Heroin

WHAT IS IT?

A derivative of morphine and thus of opium. Chemically, 3,6-O-diacetylmorphine hydrochloride monohydrate, or 'diamorphine', heroin is an almost white, crystalline, odourless powder with a bitter taste, which is rapidly and completely absorbed into the body after oral administration and is quickly distributed to all parts. In pregnant

The name was given by the developers, euphoric over their expectation of its heroic achievements in medicine. This euphoria was premature and the drug was soon found to be too addictive for general medical use. It is now the chief, and most dangerous, drug of abuse and is widely available in all 'civilized' countries. The effects for which it is taken are no more pleasant or remarkable than those of other 'recreational' drugs, but heroin rapidly leads to addiction, after which all considerations of legality, morality, justice or self-respect tend to become secondary to the pressing necessity to obtain continuing supplies. This situation is exploited by the cynical and conscienceless, who see in it an assured source of income. Addicts will lie, steal, embezzle, prostitute themselves, even murder, to get the drug or the money to buy it.

women it crosses the placenta to the fetus and causes respiratory depression and drug dependence in the newborn – a dependence which is subsequently increased if the woman breastfeeds as the drug is also excreted in the milk.

The manufacture of heroin, even for medical purposes, is illegal in almost every part of the world, except in Britain, for the drug has no medical advantages, as a pain-killer, over safer substances, except that it is more soluble than morphine so repeated injections can be avoided in terminal-care patients.

Heroin is completely converted to morphine in the body and has no medical value apart from the relief of pain of body and mind.

RISKS
Heroin, considered purely as a pharmacological agent, is not particularly likely to damage health. It is, however, in other respects, extremely likely to do so. It is easy to take a dangerous or fatal dose; the associated dangers of casual intravenous use – infection with bacteria, fungi, and various viruses including those causing AIDS and hepatitis B – are obvious; and the effects on behaviour can have devastating and destructive consequences.

HEROIN ADDICTION TREATMENT

The synthetic narcotic methadone is prescribed in a clinic and is taken by mouth in orange juice, once a day. Methadone is addictive, but does not produce a heroin 'high' and it blocks the brain-opiate receptors so that heroin, even if injected, has little effect. The supply of methadone is secure and is not dependent on criminal associations. The people under treatment may thus, although remaining addicted to methadone, lead a fairly normal life.

Some people come to prefer methadone to heroin and it is clear that many comply with the programme without any real intention of freeing themselves from the habit. Some use the methadone facilities only when heroin supplies are hard to get. Early reports of the success of the method were unduly sanguine and it has become increasingly clear that the solution to the heroin drug problem is not to be so easily found.

As with many other behavioural and criminal trends, the mere passage of time seems to bring improvement to the individual. The real reason for this is that drug-taking is the result of the failure to understand the factors which lead to satisfaction in life. The quality of early parental influence – which is vitally important in early programming – often leaves much to be desired, as may the later influence of school teachers.

But life, itself, will often, in the end, supply the deficit, and the adolescent junkie will often turn into the respectable, and disapproving, adult.

HEROIN BABIES

Heroin converts to morphine soon after entering the body and morphine in the mother's blood passes through the placenta into the blood of the fetus. Seventy-five per cent of babies born to addicted mothers show withdrawal signs and most require treatment.

RECOGNITION AND SYMPTOMS

The signs include tremor, hyperactivity, fever, vomiting, diarrhoea, sweating, sneezing, respiratory distress and convulsions. These last for an average of about a week, but sometimes persist for three weeks.

PROGNOSIS

Reports of the long-term effect on babies differ and it is difficult to separate the purely medical effects of morphine from the high level of socially disadvantageous factors in heroin addicts.

In one series, for instance, only one-quarter of the mothers were married or were living in a stable relationship. Another study, from the United States, showed a baby mortality rate, within a few weeks of birth, of nearly 7 per cent. But this may well have been because of social rather than drug-related factors and there is no real evidence that morphine, by itself, has a major influence on the health of these babies.

Hallucinogenic drugs

WHAT ARE THEY?

Psychedelic drugs derived from plants have been used for centuries because of their effect on consciousness. They have featured in religious rites, have helped to elevate the status of the medicine man, or have been used simply for recreation and for a relief from the hardships of life. Among those used are the desert cactus, *Lophophora williamsii*, known in Spanish as peyote, from which mescaline is derived; 'sacred mushrooms' of the genus Psilocybe, which contain psilocybin; the leguminous plants *Piptadenia peregrina* and *Virola calophylla*, which contain dymethyltryptamine; and the seeds of the morning glory flower, which contains lysergic acid.

In more recent years, many synthetically produced substances have been used for similar purposes but, today, in the West, the applications are almost wholly 'recreational'.

HOW THEY WORK

The study of hallucinogenic drugs and their action on the nervous system has been valuable in promoting knowledge of psychopharmacology. One of the important neuro-transmitters in the brain is serotonin (5-HT), and it is thought that hallucinogens, some of which are chemically related to serotonin, may interfere with its normal action on brain receptor sites. Although important in research, they have found little or no application in medical treatment.

EFFECTS

Among the drugs in common use are lysergic acid diethylamide (LSD), mescaline and psilocybin. A small dose of these drugs causes a sense of well-being and a heightened sensitivity to, and conviction of the significance of, all sensations and perceptions. This is followed by perceptual distortion, with vivid visual imagery and visual hallucinations. There is intensification of the emotions and modification of the emotional content so that the subject may experience anything from intense euphoria to the deepest apathy. There is an illusory, but often very strong, conviction of omniscience and of the ability to analyse and comprehend transcendental matters. Often there is a sense of expanding consciousness and a feeling of union with nature or God, accompanied by ecstasy and beatitude. Conversely, the experience may be one of terror and distress, with a sense of impending death.

The effects, of course, vary with the inclinations, stability and mental resources of the individual. Hallucinogenic drugs cannot confer data not already held and the notion that the hallucinogenic experience represents a kind of ultimate reality is nonsense. Some reactions are schizophrenic in type and these drugs may actually precipitate a frank psychotic illness in the predisposed.

Marijuana

A drug obtained from various species of the hemp grass cannabis, especially *Cannabis sativa*, *Cannabis indica* and *Cannabis americana*. The drug is widely used and has a variety of names in different parts of the world.

These include, pot, weed, grass, reefer, hashish, hash, bhang, ganja, kif and dagga. Interestingly, the word 'assassin' derives from the arabic *hashshashin* – 'a hashish eater', the story being that murderers used hash to give them courage.

EFFECTS

Cannabis resin contains many active substances, but the one which causes the desired effects is

The effects on the cardiovascular system can be dangerous and have precipitated angina pectoris, heart failure and even death in predisposed individuals. In those not habituated, it can produce panic attacks or acute anxiety and has often precipitated schizophrenia, mania, or a confusional psychosis. A state of depersonalization may also be precipitated by the drug.

tetrahydrocannabinol – one of the cannabinoids. Tetrahydrocannabinol causes widening (dilatation) of blood vessels, seen most obviously in the reddened eyes of the cannabis taker, and a fall in blood pressure. There is mild engorgement of the genitals and the heart rate increases.

PLEASURABLE PROPERTIES

The properties of tetrahydrocannabinol have long been exploited for recreational purposes, and they are widely known to recent generations in the West. They are also known for their variability, this being the result of the variety and range of different properties of the many substances present.

The main effect is euphoria – the easy promotion of laughter or giggling, often for reasons that seem silly or childish to the observer. Under the influence of the tetrahydrocannabinol there is an apparent heightening of all the senses, especially vision. Colour intensity and contrast are increased, and there is distortion of the dimensions of objects and of the perception of distance.

The perception of time, too, is distorted, or sometimes seemingly eliminated. Usually, passage of time is experienced as being slower than reality, so that estimates of periods past are greater than clock time and of future periods less. One of the much-valued properties among some devotees is the sense of deep philosophical insight conveyed by the cannabinoids. There is a conviction of omniscience, of knowing all the answers to the riddles of the universe, and this is often accompanied by a feeling of calm superiority, so that one hardly bothers to bring the great accessible truths to mind.

For those of genuine philosophical bent, however, the inability to retain these insights, as the effects of the drug wear off, is a bitter disappointment. This particular effect is not specific to this group of drugs and is often experienced, for instance, during recovery from a short anaesthetic. The effect is, of course, an illusion. In fact, intellectual performance is impaired during the period of the drug action.

Mental arithmetic is less accurate than normal and short-term memory defective. The affected person often forgets the beginning of a sentence before reaching the end.

PERFORMANCE

The effects on performance should be known. Slowing of reflexes, distortion of distance and alteration in the sense of responsibility all have a serious effect on skilled activities such as driving, patient monitoring, air traffic controlling, military surveillance, etc., and it is right that the public should be protected against the use of cannabis by people engaged in these activities. There is little evidence that cannabis promotes criminal activity.

BRAIN DAMAGE

Controversy continues in medical circles as to whether the cannabinoids cause organic brain damage. This has been positively demonstrated in rats and monkeys, but not objectively in humans. Neither CT scanning nor electroencephalography have shown changes.

There is, however, plenty of indirect evidence of brain dysfunction in persistent heavy users. Such people can develop the amotivational syndrome and show apathy and loss of interest and concern. Students stop working, suffer a drop in academic performance and give up courses.

This effect is to be expected because the cannabinoids are concentrated in the limbic system, which is the motivational centre of the brain and because of the effects on memory and reasoning.

Drug interaction with the cannabinoids is important. It has been shown that cannabis interferes with certain liver enzymes necessary for the breakdown of some drugs.

One consequence is that the effect of medicinal drugs may be unexpectedly and dangerously prolonged. Barbiturates, for instance, keep one asleep longer if taken after cannabis has been used.

Cannabinoids have been shown to cause damage to chromosomes and impairment of cell division and readily cause fetal abnormalities in animals in dosage equivalent to that commonly used in man. Happily, there has, so far, been no sign of inherited genetic defects, or thalidomide-like effects, in humans, but it seems likely that cannabis is causing an increase in the rate of early spontaneous abortion.

WITHDRAWAL

Cannabis withdrawal produces quite severe symptoms, including anxiety, irritability, headaches, sleeplessness, muscle twitching, sweating and diarrhoea, but these will pass and, in most cases, the amotivational syndrome will eventually resolve.

PROGRESSION TO HARDER DRUGS

Concern has been expressed about the probability of progress from cannabis use to that of harder drugs. Only a small proportion of casual users do progress, but it is clear that heavy users commonly do progress.

Nearly all heroin addicts have had previous experience of cannabis. It is unnecessary to propose any pharmacological reason for this, but undoubtedly the cannabis experience in certain predisposed individuals does, for psychological reasons, cause progression to drugs such as heroin. This was accepted by the Canadian Commission of Inquiry into the Non-Medical Use of Drugs, in their 1972 report on cannabis.

Solvent abuse

The deliberate inhalation of the vapour from various solvents for the sake of their narcotic effect. Substances used in this way include any of the solvent-based commercial adhesives, volatile cleaning fluids, lighter fuel, petrol, paint thinner solvents, marking ink, anti-freeze, nail varnish remover, butane gas and toluene. Usually, a small quantity of the solvent is poured into a polythene bag which is held tightly against the nose and mouth, so as to exclude additional air and avoid reducing the vapour concentration.

The effects vary, but are generally intoxicant, with loss of full awareness of the surroundings, incoordination and loss of muscle control and, sometimes, hallucinations. Unconsciousness may occur and episodes can end fatally, usually by asphyxiation, inhalation of vomit, or accident.

The practice is often performed in groups and many youngsters take to it as a result of peer pressure. While, for many, glue sniffing episodes are merely experimental and of little importance, a considerable number of tragic deaths have resulted from this dangerous practice. Children should be clearly informed of the risks.

Many reports have been published of brain, liver and kidney damage from solvent abuse. Addiction can occur and habituation is rapid so that ever larger doses are required to produce the desired effect. These large doses are liable to cause organ damage.

Detecting suspected drug abuse in young people

Without direct evidence in the form of actual drug possession or the finding of drug equipment among the young person's belongings, it is seldom that anyone can be quite sure that a young person is abusing drugs. There are, however, several indicators that should arouse strong suspicion. Remember that the maintenance of a drug habit is expensive and that the young person has to get money from somewhere. Warning signs, that should never be ignored, include:

◆ unexplained losses of money or valuables from the household;
◆ possession by the young person of unexplained sums of money;
◆ secretive behaviour;

◆ apparent personality changes or mood swings;

◆ deterioration in personal appearance;

◆ sudden reduction in school/college performance;

◆ loss of interest in former activities such as sport;

◆ acquisition of new acquaintances and rejection of old friends;

◆ inability to account for activities during regular periods of time;

◆ memory loss;

◆ accident proneness.

Many young people, unable to obtain the money they need for drugs, turn to drug-dealing. In this case, they may have more money than can plausibly be accounted for. However, most of these signs may have an innocent explanation. Schizophrenia and other psychiatric disturbances commonly develop during adolescence, and this is also a period when young people may have severe, but often temporary, behaviour problems. An aggressive response to these is inappropriate and unproductive and a major effort at sympathy and understanding is often required of older people. It may often be best to discuss openly the possibility of drug abuse.

A note about laetrile

A drug obtained from bitter almonds, apricot seeds and the seeds of other fruit, which has been claimed to be of value in the treatment of cancer. The drug is said to be broken down in the body to yield a cyanide-containing compound called mandelonitrile. The breakdown to this substance is effected by enzymes called beta glucosidases and it is claimed that more cyanide is released in the region of cancer cells than elsewhere because cancer cells contain more beta glucosidases than healthy tissues. It is also claimed that cancers are less able than normal tissues to break down the toxic cyanide compound to a non-toxic form.

Unfortunately, careful study of the reports of alleged successes with this drug have shown no medically acceptable evidence that laetrile has any value in the treatment of cancer. Individual case reports have been over-optimistic, lacking in scientific controls and follow-up, and based on subjective, rather than objective, criteria. As a result of these reports, however, the hopes of many cancer sufferers have been unjustifiably raised and the issue has, understandably, become highly emotional and controversial.

A to Z
of Drugs
and
Drug Actions

TThis dictionary contains most of the important drugs in use today, entered under both generic names and trade names. It also includes the main drug groups with an account of their actions and uses.

Considerations of space preclude full explanations of all diseases and medical concepts mentioned.

Trade names are capitalized. Generic drug names and, with a few exceptions, drug groups, have a lower case initial letter. Drugs, drug groups, terms and preparations set all in capitals are referred to elsewhere in this section, under that name.

KEY

The symbol **[O]** indicates that the drug is either available over-the-counter or that an over-the-counter drug with the same active ingredient or ingredients is available.

The symbol **[»]** indicates the forms in which the drug can be taken.

The symbol **[S]** sets out side-effects.

The symbol **[W]** indicates a drug recently withdrawn. These drugs should not be used.

Abdec
a trade name for a multivitamin preparation. **[O]**

ACE inhibitors
See ANGIOTENSIN-CONVERTING ENZYME INHIBITORS.

acebutolol
a beta-blocker drug commonly used to treat high blood pressure and angina. A trade name is Sectral.

acedapsone
a drug used to treat leprosy.

Acepril
a trade name for CAPTOPRIL.

acetaminophen
a generic drug name derived from acetanilide and widely used as the proprietary drug Panadol (PARACETAMOL) to relieve pain and reduce fever.

[S] *The drug does not irritate the stomach, as ASPIRIN does, but overdose causes liver and kidney damage and may cause death from liver failure. Fifteen grams or more is potentially serious. The victim remains well for a day or two and liver failure develops between the third and fifth day.*

Other trade names are Anacin-3, Tempra and Tylenol. **[0]**

acetazolamide
a carbonic anhydrase inhibitor diuretic drug used in the treatment of glaucoma when the intraocular

pressure rise cannot be controlled with eyedrops alone. A trade name is Diamox.

acetohexamide
a drug of the sulphonylurea group used to treat Type II (maturity-onset) diabetes. A trade name is Dymelor.

Acetopt
a trade name for eye drops containing SULPHACETAMIDE.

acetylcysteine
a drug used to reduce the stickiness and viscosity of mucus. A mucolytic. It is useful for freeing sputum in bronchitis and in liquefying mucus in cystic fibrosis. It is also used to improve eye comfort in keratoconjunctivitis sicca. A trade name is Mucomyst.

acetylsalicylic acid
the common analgesic and antiprostaglandin drug Aspirin. [0]

Achromycin
a trade name for TETRACYCLINE.

Achrostatin
a trade name for TETRACYCLINE and NYSTATIN.

aclarubicin
an antimitotic (anticancer) drug administered by
injection. A trade name is Aclacin.

Acnacyl
a trade name for BENZOYL PEROXIDE.

Acnegel
a trade name for BENZOYL PEROXIDE.

acriflavine
a powder derived from acridine and used, in
solution, as an antiseptic for skin cleansing and
wound irrigation.

acrivastine
an ANTIHISTAMINE drug used to treat hay fever
and urticaria. A trade name is Semprex.

Actacode
a trade name for CODEINE.

ACTH
adrenocorticotropic hormone. This hormone is produced by the pituitary gland, on instructions from the hypothalamus when a stressful situation arises. ACTH is carried by the blood to the adrenal glands and prompts them to secrete the hormone cortisol into the bloodstream. ACTH is sometimes used as a drug to promote this effect.

Acthar
a trade name for ACTH.

Actifed
a trade name for TRIPROLIDINE and PSEUDOEPHEDRINE. [0]

Actilyse
a trade name for TISSUE PLASMINOGEN ACTIVATOR.

actinomycin
an ANTIBIOTIC which causes breaks in DNA. This
side effect renders it unsuitable as an antibacterial
drug, but makes it useful as an anticancer drug.

activated charcoal
a highly absorbent form of carbon used to absorb
gas, to deodorize and to inactivate a number of
ingested poisons.

Actraphane
a trade name for INSULIN.

Actrapid
a trade name for INSULIN.

Actuss
a trade name for PHOLCODINE.

Acupan
a trade name for nefopam, a non-narcotic
ANALGESIC.

acyclovir

a drug highly active against the Herpes simplex
virus and against the closely similar varicella-zoster
virus which causes chickenpox and shingles. Early
treatment with the drug, taken by mouth, can
greatly reduce the severity of shingles. Acyclovir is
widely used to treat genital herpes and, although it
cannot cure this condition, it can greatly reduce its
severity. A trade name is Zovirax. [O]

Adalat

a trade name for NIFEDIPINE.

Adriamycin

doxorubicin. An anticancer drug which acts by
interfering with cell division.

Adroyd

a trade name for OXYMETHOLONE.

albendazole

a drug used to get rid of roundworms, hookworms
and other worm parasites. A trade name is
Eskazole.

Albustix
a trade name for a urine dip strip test for albumin.

alclometasone
a CORTICOSTEROID DRUG administered externally
as a cream or ointment to treat inflammatory skin
disorders. A trade name is Modrasone.

Alclox
a trade name for CLOXACILLIN.

Alcobon
a trade name for FLUCYTOSINE.

Alcopar
a trade name for BEPHENIUM.

alcuronium
a neuro-muscular junction blocking drug causing
profound muscle relaxation. It is used by
anaesthetists and administered by injection. A
trade name is Alloferin.

Aldactone
a trade name for SPIRONOLACTONE.

Aldazine
a trade name for THIORIDAZINE.

Aldecin
a trade name for BECLOMETHASONE.

aldesleukin
human interleukin (interleukin-2) produced by
recombinant DNA technology (genetic
engineering). Interleukins act to enhance the
function of the immune system. Aldesleukin
prompts T lymphocytes to become cytotoxic (killer)
cells, active against cancer cells. The results against
certain cancers such as melanomas or kidney cell
cancer have been encouraging. A trade name is
Proleukin.

Aldomet
a trade name for methyldopa, a powerful
ANTIHYPERSENSITIVE drug.

KEY

The symbol **[O]** indicates that the drug is either available over-the-counter or that an over-the-counter drug with the same active ingredient or ingredients is available.

The symbol **[»]** indicates the forms in which the drug can be taken.

The symbol **[S]** sets out side-effects.

The symbol **[W]** indicates a drug recently withdrawn. These drugs should not be used.

Alepam

a trade name for OXAZEPAM.

alfacalcidol

a synthetic form of vitamin D used to treat low blood calcium and bone softening (osteomalacia) caused by kidney disease. A trade name is One-alpha.

alfentanil hydrochloride
a narcotic ANALGESIC drug used to relieve severe pain. A trade name is Rapifen.

Algicon
a trade name for a mixture of antacid drugs.

alginic acid
an antacid drug used to treat heartburn caused by acid reflux into the gullet and hiatus hernia. A trade name is Gastrocote, Gastron.

Alkeran
a trade name for MELPHALAN.

Alleract
a trade name for TRIPROLIDINE and PSEUDOEPHEDRINE. [0]

Aller-eze
a trade name for CLEMASTINE. [0]

allopurinol
a drug used to treat gout. Allopurinol is a xanthine

oxidase inhibitor which reduces the production of uric acid from nucleic acid breakdown. Trade names are Aloral, Aluline, Caplenal, Cosuric, Hamarin Lopurin, Zyloprim and Zyloric.

Allormed
a trade name for ALLOPURINOL.

Almacarb
a trade name for a mixture of ALUMINIUM HYDROXIDE and MAGNESIUM CARBONATE. [0]

Almodan
a trade name for AMOXICILLIN.

Alodorm
a trade name for NITRAZEPAM.

aloin
a mild laxative used in proprietary constipation remedies. A trade name in Alophen. [0]

Aloral
a trade name for ALLOPURINOL.

aloxiprin
a non-steroidal pain-killing and anti-inflammatory
drug (NSAID).

alpha-adrenergic blocker
one of a group of drugs that can occupy alpha-
adrenoceptor sites on arteries, so blocking the
action of adrenaline-like hormones and causing
widening of arteries (vasodilatation) and a drop in
the blood pressure. They include prazosin,
doxazocin, tolazoline, indoramin,
phenoxybenzamine and thymoxamine.

[S] *Overdosage causes a severe drop in blood
pressure, a fast pulse, nausea, vomiting and
diarrhoea, a dry mouth, flushed skin, convulsions,
drowsiness and coma.*

Alphamox
a trade name for AMOXICILLIN.

alphatocopherol
vitamin E.

Alphosyl

a trade name for allantoin and COAL TAR, a preparation used in the treatment of psoriasis.

Alprim

a trade name for TRIMETHOPRIM.

alprostadil

a prostaglandin drug administered by injection to improve lung blood flow in newborn babies with congenital heart defects who are awaiting surgery. A trade name is Prostin VR.

alteplase

a TISSUE PLASMINOGEN ACTIVATOR drug made by recombinant DNA technology. The drug is used to dissolve blood clots in the circulation, especially in the coronary arteries of the heart. A trade name is Actilyse.

Aludrox

a trade name for ALUMINIUM HYDROXIDE. **[0]**

Aluline

a trade name for ALLOPURINOL.

aluminium hydroxide

an antacid drug. Trade names are Alu-cap, Aludrox, Alu-Tab, Amphojel and Dialume. **[0]**

Alupent

a trade name for orciprenaline.

Alupram

a trade name for DIAZEPAM.

alverine citrate

a bulking agent and antispasmodic drug used to treat the irritable bowel syndrome and other colonic disorders. Trade names are Alvercol, or Spasmonal.

amantadine

an antiviral drug, also used to treat Parkinson's disease. A trade name is Symmetrel.

amethocaine
a local anaesthetic drug which is effective when in contact with surfaces as well as when given by injection.

[S] *It resembles COCAINE in its action and can readily be absorbed in dangerous amounts from mucous membranes.*

A trade name is Anethaine.

Amfipen
a trade name for AMPICILLIN.

amidopyrine
aminopyrine. A pain-killing drug once widely used as an aspirin substitute. It's now out of favour because of the risk of inducing a sometimes fatal drop in the number of white cells in the blood (agranulocytosis).

amikacin
an ANTIBIOTIC drug, one of the AMINOGLYCOSIDES.

amiloride

a non-steroidal DIURETIC drug that acts by reducing reabsorption of sodium, and thus water, in the kidneys. A 'potassium-sparing' diuretic. A trade name is Midamor.

aminocaproic acid

a drug that reduces the tendency for fibrin in the blood to be broken down. It thus aids in the clotting of blood in wounds.

aminoglutethimide

a drug that interferes with the synthesis of STEROIDS, OESTROGENS and ANDROGENS by the adrenal glands. It does this by blocking an enzyme that allows the conversion of cholesterol.

aminoglycosides

a class of antibiotics which include STREPTOMYCIN, TOBRAMYCIN, KANAMYCIN, AMIKACIN, GENTAMICIN and NEOMYCIN. They act by causing misreading of certain codons on messenger RNA and are transported into bacterial cells only if free oxygen is present.

[S] *The aminoglycosides can cause deafness and tinnitus if taken in excess or if not excreted normally because of kidney disease.*

[S] *They can also cause damage to the kidneys.*

aminophylline
a drug used in the control of asthma. In acute cases it can be given by intravenous injection but it is also effective by mouth or in a suppository.

amiodarone
a drug used to control abnormal heart rhythms such as fibrillation of the upper chambers (atrial fibrillation) or abnormally rapid heartbeat. A trade name is Cordarone X.

Amitrip
a trade name for AMITRIPTYLINE.

amitriptyline
a tricyclic ANTIDEPRESSANT drug. Trade names are Domical, Elavil, Lentizol and Tryptizol.

amlodipine
a calcium antagonist drug used to treat angina pectoris. A trade name is Istin.

amodiaquine
an antimalarial drug used in the event of QUININE intolerance in CHLOROQUINE-resistant Plasmodium falciparum malaria.

amoebicide
a drug used to kill pathogenic amoebae.

amorolfine
an antimycotic drug administered as a cream for external use for the treatment of tinea, candidiasis and other skin fungus infections and for tinea of the nails. A trade name is Loceryl.

amoxapine
a tricyclic ANTIDEPRESSANT drug similar to IMIPRAMINE.

[S] *Overdosage may cause acute kidney failure, convulsions and coma.* A trade name is Asendis.

amoxicillin

an ampicillin-like penicillin ANTIBIOTIC, effective in
TYPHOID and many other infections. A trade name
is Amoxil.

Amoxidin

a trade name for AMOXICILLIN.

Amoxil

a trade name for AMOXICILLIN.

amphetamine

a central nervous system (CNS) stimulant drug with
few medical uses but commonly abused to obtain a
'high'.

[S] *Amphetamine use leads to tolerance and
sometimes physical dependence.*

[S] *Overdosage causes irritability, tremor,
restlessness, insomnia, flushing, nausea and
vomiting, irregularity of the pulse, delirium,
hallucinations, convulsions and coma.*

[S] *Amphetamine can precipitate a psychosis in predisposed people.*

Amphogel
a trade name for ALUMINIUM HYDROXIDE. **[O]**

amphotericin-B
an ANTIBIOTIC drug used to treat fungus infections within the body.

KEY

The symbol **[O]** indicates that the drug is either available over-the-counter or that an over-the-counter drug with the same active ingredient or ingredients is available.

The symbol **[»]** indicates the forms in which the drug can be taken.

The symbol **[S]** sets out side-effects.

The symbol **[W]** indicates a drug recently withdrawn. These drugs should not be used.

[S] *It is moderately toxic and side-effects are common.*

A trade name is Fungilin.

ampicillin
a widely used penicillin ANTIBIOTIC, effective by mouth and capable of killing many gram-negative as well as gram-positive organisms. About one-third of the dose is excreted unchanged in the urine.

[S] *The drug precipitates a characteristic rash if given to people incubating glandular fever (infective mononucleosis).*

A trade name is Penbritin.

Amprace
a trade name for ENALAPRIL.

amsacrine
a cytotoxic anticancer drug administered by injection. A trade name is Amsidine.

amyl nitrite
a volatile drug used by inhalation in the control of pain in angina pectoris. It acts by relaxing smooth muscle and thus dilating arteries, including the coronary arteries. The pain is relieved because of the improved blood supply to the heart muscle.

Amytal
a trade name for amylobarbitone, a barbiturate hypnotic drug of medium duration of action.

anabolic steroids
drugs that cause tissue growth by stimulating protein synthesis. They are synthetic male sex hormone steroids such as ethyloestrenol, methandrenone, nandrolone, norethandrolone, oxymesterone and stanolone. Their use may sometimes be justified to help elderly and underweight people to gain strength and they can be valuable in osteoporosis.

[S] *Anabolic steroids have been widely used by body-building enthusiasts and athletes to improve muscle bulk and strength. This has rightly been* *declared illegal, not only because of its intrinsic unfairness to other competitors, but also because of the possible adverse effects on health.*

[S] *Among other health disorders, anabolic steroids can cause a dangerous form of enlargement of the heart and can precipitate serious psychiatric effects. These include major depression, hallucinations, religious delusions, 'thought-broadcasting', paranoid jealousy, delusions of grandeur and manic behaviour.*

anaesthetic drugs
drugs used to allow painless surgery,with or without loss of consciousness. Narcotic drugs, such as morphine, omnopon or Valium (diazepam), are used before an operation (pre-medication), to promote confidence, relax muscles and help the patient to forget the unpleasantness afterwards. The drug atropine is often given to reduce the tendency for fluid to collect in the air tubes.

Nowadays, general anaesthesia is almost always induced by a small injection into a vein of a rapid-acting drug, such as the barbiturate Pentothal (thiopentone). This is very pleasant and there is hardly any awareness of what is happening. Anaesthesia is maintained, at a very light level for safety, by means of inhaled drugs such as nitrous oxide or halothane. These are often combined with a strong pain-killing (ANALGESIC) drug because, although the person concerned is unconscious, stimuli which would otherwise be painful can still cause unwanted changes in the body.

If muscle relaxation is needed, this is now achieved by one of a number of drugs which temporarily paralyse the muscles. In this event, the breathing must be maintained artificially. Sometimes the blood pressure is deliberately lowered by ANTIHYPERTENSIVE DRUGS.

Local anaesthetic drugs act in the vicinity of nerves by blocking the passage of nerve impulses. So, if the nerves concerned are those which would carry pain impulses to the brain, no pain will be felt. The area affected by the local anaesthetic will have be unpleasantly numb, for the duration of the action of the drug.

[»] *They are mostly used for minor surgical and dental operations and can be given by injection into, or around, the area to be operated upon, or sometimes by simple application to the surface. They are also given in the form of eye drops, anaesthetic throat sprays, anaesthetic nasal packs and lozenges to be sucked.*

Sometimes it is safer and more convenient to use the local anaesthetic to block the nerves carrying the sensation, at a point remote from the operation site. Assuming all sensory nerves from the area are blocked, the effect is exactly the same. The nerve block can be made at a point near the operation site – as in the common mandibular dental block, which anaesthetizes half of the jaw and lower lip or it may be made further away, as in spinal, epidural and pudendal block anaesthetics. In all cases the principle is the same.

While removing all pain sensation, local anaesthetics do not necessarily remove all sensation. In a vasectomy operation, for instance, one may experience an odd grating, or vibrating, feeling as some of the tissues are cut. This kind of sensation results from the transmission of sound-like vibrations, through the tissues, to nerves which are not anaesthetized.

Local anaesthetics begin to act as soon as they are injected and the anaesthetic effect is usually full within about five minutes. Their duration of action depends on the drug used – there is a wide range of local anaesthetics – and may be as long as four hours from a single injection. Shorter-acting anaesthetics are often prevented from dispersing by adding adrenaline which constricts blood vessels and prolongs the action of the anaesthetic.

Anafranil
a trade name for CLOMIPRAMINE.

analeptic drugs
drugs which stimulate the nerve centres in the brain responsible for breathing. Their action is to increase the strength of the output, from the brain,

of the nerve impulses to the respiratory muscles –
the diaphragm and the muscles between the ribs
(intercostal muscles). Analeptics, such as doxapram
or nikethamide are used to stimulate absent
breathing (apnoea) in newborn babies and are
sometimes used in cases of respiratory failure from
drug overdose or to speed recovery from a general
anaesthetic. The drug naloxone, which is an
antagonist to opiate drugs, while not an analeptic,
is commonly used in such cases.

analgesic drugs
the important group of pain-killing drugs. It
includes a wide range of drugs from the mild and
comparatively safe, such as paracetamol, to the
powerful and dangerous, such as the narcotic
drugs.

Paracetamol works mainly by blocking the passage
of the nerve impulses for pain so that they do not
reach the part of the brain where pain is perceived.
Most of the other mild analgesics, such as aspirin
and the non-steroidal anti-inflammatory drugs
(NSAIDs), work in a different way. When tissue cells

are injured in any way – either by mechanical force, bacterial poisons or other causes of inflammation – they release powerful substances called prostaglandins. Prostaglandins strongly stimulate pain nerve endings and the result is the experience of pain. NSAIDs act by blocking the production of prostaglandins. NSAIDs include such drugs as ibuprofen, fenoprofen, naproxen and mefenamic acid.

Drugs like morphine act on the brain; others act on nerve conduction. But the aspirin-like drugs act directly on damaged cells and work solely by preventing the production of the substances which cause the pain. Aspirin has no effect on the pain of a needle-prick because this directly stimulates the pain nerve endings. Nor has it any effect on the pain caused by an injection of prostaglandins.

[S] *Aspirin has a bad reputation for causing irritation to the lining of the stomach. A plain aspirin tablet kept between gum and cheek for half an hour will turn the mucous membrane white and wrinkled and will loosen the surface. Aspirin*

KEY

The symbol **[O]** indicates that the drug is either available over-the-counter or that an over-the-counter drug with the same active ingredient or ingredients is available.

The symbol **[»]** indicates the forms in which the drug can be taken.

The symbol **[S]** sets out side-effects.

The symbol **[W]** indicates a drug recently withdrawn. These drugs should not be used.

---

can do the same to the stomach lining causing congestion and bleeding around undissolved particles.

[S] *Over half of all people taking aspirin have traces of blood in their stools. So plain aspirin should never be used. Only the soluble variety, which greatly reduces the danger, is safe. People with indigestion or a previous history of ulcer trouble should never take aspirin.*

[S] *Following a virus infection in children, aspirin can cause the serious liver and brain disorder Reye's syndrome. It is no longer given to children.*

[S] *Aspirin hypersensitivity, especially in people with other allergies, is rare, but can cause alarming and often dangerous reactions, including severe breathing difficulty.*

[S] *Aspirin and the NSAIDs cause prolongation of the bleeding time. This can sometimes be dangerous. A minor eye injury with a small leak of blood into the front chamber can be turned into a massive intra-ocular haemorrhage by a single aspirin tablet, which doubles the bleeding time for up to a week.*

[S] *Paracetamol is a serious liver poison if many tablets are taken at once. Twenty tablets can cause severe liver damage. The antidote is methionine.*

An intermediate group of analgesics consists of a mixture of these mild analgesics with the mild – and fairly safe – narcotic analgesic, codeine. There is a large range of proprietary medications consisting of various combinations of codeine, aspirin and various NSAIDs. Other moderately potent narcotic drugs, unlikely to cause addiction, are dihydrocodeine, pentazocine and dextropropoxyphene.

For the relief of very severe pain, more powerful narcotic drugs may be needed. These are used only when other drugs are ineffective, and include morphine, phenazocine and methadone. The narcotic analgesics act on specific receptor sites, called opiate receptors, in the brain and spinal cord, blocking the pain sensation. The natural endorphins of the body act in the same way. These strong narcotic analgesics also produce a powerful feeling of well-being (euphoria) and are abused for this reason.

[S] *They are strongly addictive. Heroin (diamorphine), formerly widely used in medicine, is now banned in most countries because of this danger.*

Anamorph

a trade name for morphine.

Anapolon

a trade name for OXYMETHOLONE.

Anatensol

a trade name for FLUPHENAZINE.

Ancolan

a trade name for MECLOZINE.

Ancoloxin

a trade name for MECLOZINE.

Ancotil

a trade name for FLUCYTOSINE.

Andriol

a trade name for TESTOSTERONE.

androgens

male sex hormones. Androgens are STEROIDS and
include testosterone and androsterone. As drugs,

they are used to stimulate the development of
sexual characteristics in boys when there is
inadequate output from the testicles and to
stimulate red cell formation in aplastic anaemia.
See also ANABOLIC STEROIDS. The term androgen
derives from the Greek andros, a man and gennao,
to make.

Andrumin
a trade name for DIMENHYDRINATE.

Anethaine
a trade name for AMETHOCAINE.

angel dust
a slang term for the powerful ANALGESIC and
anaesthetic drug Phencyclidine commonly abused
for recreational purposes. It is also known by the
abbreviation PCP.

*Abuse of this drug can lead to muscle rigidity,
convulsions and death.*

Angilol
a trade name for PROPRANOLOL.

Anginine
a trade name for GLYCERYL TRINITRATE.

angiotensin-converting enzyme inhibitors
a class of drugs used in the treatment of raised
blood pressure. They act by interfering with the
action of the enzyme that converts the inactive
angiotensin I to the powerful artery constrictor
angiotensin II. The absence of this substance allows
arteries to widen and the blood pressure to drop.

[»] *They are administered by mouth.*

Trade names are Captopril, Enalapril.

anistreplase
a drug consisting of a complex of the clot-
dissolving substances streptokinase and
plasminogen. It is used to dissolve blood clots in the
circulation. A trade name is Eminase.

anorectic drugs
drugs that suppress appetite and may be useful in the management of obesity. They include AMPHETAMINE and its derivatives, diethylpropion (Tenuate), mazindol (Teronc) and fenfluramine (Ponderax).

Anpec
a trade name for VERAPAMIL.

Antabuse
disulfiram. A drug sometimes used in the management of alcoholism, which causes severe nausea and vomiting, sweating, breathlessness, headache and chest pain if any alcohol is taken after it has been given. Disulfiram inhibits the enzyme that breaks down acetaldehyde, a toxic metabolite of alcohol, so that this accumulates. The method is a form of aversion therapy and is not without danger of collapse and death from the toxic effects.

antacid drugs
drugs used to reduce or neutralize excess stomach

acid and to relieve the symptoms of heartburn (acid reflux).

Stomach and duodenal ulcers (peptic ulcers) are caused by the action of stomach acid and the protein-splitting enzyme, pepsin, on the lining of the bowel. Pepsin only works in the presence of acid. The stomach lining is normally protected by a layer of mucus, secreted by many cells in the lining. Any defect in this mucous layer allows the stomach contents to start digesting the wall. Smoking and the over-use of irritating drugs like strong alcohol, aspirin and brufen are among the causes of such a defect. The more acid present the more likely is self-digestion to occur.

The part of the bowel immediately beyond the stomach (the duodenum) contains alkaline secretions which tend to neutralize the stomach acid. So duodenal ulcers only occur if there is excess of acid and pepsin. If the acid levels can be kept low enough neither stomach nor duodenal ulcers will occur. This can be done in two ways – by preventing the acid from being produced by the use of drugs such as cimetidine or ranitidine, or by chemically neutralizing the acid once it has been produced. The drugs which do this are called antacids.

The most popular and cheapest antacid is the alkali baking soda (sodium bicarbonate). This acts quickly and gives rapid relief of pain but the reaction with the acid results in the production of large volumes of carbon dioxide gas. Much belching results.

[S] *The bicarbonate is absorbed into the blood and excess can make the blood alkaline – which can be serious.*

Other antacids include magnesium oxide, magnesium hydroxide and magnesium trisilicate. These are not absorbed, and the first two also act as purgatives. Magnesium trisilicate works more slowly than the oxides and large doses are needed, but in addition to neutralizing the acid, it also inactivates the pepsin and is quite effective. Aludrox (aluminium hydroxide) also binds the pepsin and neutralizes the acid. It, too, must be taken in large dosage for full effect.

Like the rest of the stomach contents, antacids are quickly passed out of the stomach. About half has gone in half an hour. So it is not really satisfactory to take them only when pain is felt –as is the common practice. The management of dyspepsia and peptic ulcers involves more than just the use of antacids and self-treatment is not always safe.

See also H_2 RECEPTOR ANTAGONISTS.

antazoline
an ANTIHISTAMINE drug that also has weak local anaesthetic and ANTICHOLINERGIC effects. It is commonly used in the form of eyedrops. A trade name is Antistin-Privine.

Antenex
a trade name for DIAZEPAM.

Antepar
a trade name for PIPERAZINE.

Anthel
a trade name for PYRANTEL.

anthelmintic
a drug used to kill or drive out parasitic worms from the intestines. From the Greek anti, against and elmins, a worm. Different kinds of drugs are used to kill or paralyse different worms and it is important for the type of worm to be identified before treatment is started. The drugs used either kill or paralyse the worms, so that their attachment to the lining of the bowel, or to the tissues, is broken. The worms then pass out with the stools or may, if necessary, be removed surgically from tissues. Sometimes a laxative is given with the anthelmintic drug to help in the evacuation of intestinal worms.

Commonly used anthelmintic drugs include piperazine for roundworms and threadworms; tetrachloroethylene or thiabendazole for hookworms; niclosamide or praziquantel for tapeworms; niridazole or metronidazole for guinea worm; diethylcarbamazine for filariasis;

> **KEY**
>
> The symbol [O] indicates that the drug is either available over-the-counter or that an over-the-counter drug with the same active ingredient or ingredients is available.
>
> The symbol [»] indicates the forms in which the drug can be taken.
>
> The symbol [S] sets out side-effects.
>
> The symbol [W] indicates a drug recently withdrawn. These drugs should not be used.

praziquantel for schistosomiasis; mebendazole for whipworm; and diethylcarbamazine or thiabendazole for toxocariasis (larva migrans).

Anthisan
a trade name for mepyramine, an ANTIHISTAMINE.

Anthranol [W]
a trade name for DITHRANOL.

anti-androgen drugs

drugs given to sexually criminal men to inhibit male sex hormone action and dampen down their urges. These include cyproterone acetate, CIMETIDINE and SPIRONOLACTONE.

[S] *Anti-androgen drugs may cause breast enlargement (gynaecomastia).*

anti-anxiety drugs

drugs used to treat abnormal anxiety. Anxiety cannot be separated from the physical effects (symptoms) associated with it, such as muscle tension, tremor, sweating and a fast heart rate. Some workers even believe that these symptoms are actually the cause of the anxiety, rather than the effect. Certainly, any drug which controls these symptoms will tend to relieve the level of anxiety and may even temporarily abolish it altogether.

Anti-anxiety drugs, sometimes rather fancifully called 'anxiolytics' are, in general, minor sedatives and tranquillizers that relax muscles and slow the heart. They include beta-blockers, such as propranolol and oxprenolol, and benzodiazepines, such as Valium (diazepam) and Librium (chlordiazepoxide). Barbiturate drugs are seldom used nowadays.

Anti-anxiety drugs, although useful, are not the definitive treatment for anxiety. This must involve a study of the life problems and reactions underlying the anxiety and skilled counselling and advice by a wise psychotherapist.

anti-arrhythmic drugs
drugs used to correct irregularity of the heart beat. They include DIGOXIN, VERAPAMIL, AMIODARONE, QUINIDINE, procainamide, LIGNOCAINE, flecainide and CALCIUM CHANNEL BLOCKERS. These drugs act in different ways to convert irregular and inefficient contractions into steady, slower and more forceful beats, thereby improving the pumping efficiency of the heart.

antibiotic drugs
drugs that can kill bacteria within the body. The group of the antibiotics is one of the largest groups

of drugs and one of the best known. The benefits conferred on humanity by the antibiotics are beyond computation. Sixty years ago, medicine was dominated by bacterial infection, which was the major cause of death and was responsible for an immense amount of suffering, persistent ill-health and disability. Mothers would listen with alarm to their children's coughing or contemplate with terror red streaks running up the arm and enlarged lymph nodes. Compound fractures of limbs often led to amputation. A squeezed pustule on the nose might cause a spreading fatal infection into the brain. Lobar pneumonia was commonplace and often fatal, and osteomyelitis caused discharging channels (sinuses) for years. Tuberculosis sanitoria were full of people coughing up blood and lung tissue.

All that has changed and most people alive today have no concept of a world without antibiotics. These drugs are able to kill germs (micro-organisms) in the body, or to prevent their growth or reproduction, without killing the patient. As a result, almost all diseases caused by infecting bacteria can now be cured by antibiotics.

Note, however, that antibiotics have no effect on viruses.

Antibiotics were originally derived from cultures of living organisms, such as fungi or bacteria, but, today, many can be chemically synthesized.

There is widespread criticism of the way some doctors use antibiotics. The proponents of alternative medicine assure us that antibiotics do more harm than good and that doctors dish them out for everything. Much of this criticism is uninformed but, unfortunately, some of it is justified. Some doctors, more concerned with immediate clinical problems than with seemingly academic exhortations from the experts, prescribe them needlessly or for trivial infections.

Sometimes, this misuse stems from pressure from patients, and sometimes it occurs because busy doctors feel they cannot take chances with possibly potentially serious infections but do not have time to investigate the cases as thoroughly as they might.

Hospital doctors, understandably, are often more concerned with the immediate pressing needs of their patients than with the possible future hazards to society as a whole, and do sometimes prescribe powerful new drugs when safer, established, remedies would suffice. The two essential problems are the development of strains of bacteria resistant to antibiotics and the risk of undesirable side-effects.

If antibiotics are used casually and in inadequate dosage – and this is not always the doctor's fault – the bacteria which are very sensitive will be killed but those which, by chance, have a natural genetic resistance may survive. When these reproduce, clones of resistant organisms result. This process of natural selection is accelerated by the short bacterial generation – only about twenty minutes – in ideal conditions. As a result, many organisms are now resistant. This has put a heavy demand on the energy of research workers to produce new and better antibiotics, so as to keep ahead. So today, we have an on-going race between the development of resistance in bacteria, on the one hand, and the development of new antibiotics, on the other. We should indeed be grateful to the dedicated men and women who labour to produce new and more effective antibiotics, for it is only through their efforts that, on the whole, we keep ahead in the race.

There are many antibiotics and the proliferation of official and trade names is bewildering. But they fall into groups, the members of each of which are related chemically, or by derivation, to each other. These groups are the penicillins (penicillin G, penicillin V, cloxacillin, flucloxacillin and many others); the cephalosporins (cephaloridine, cephalothin, cefuroxime and many others); the aminoglycosides (gentamycin, streptomycin, tobramycin, netilmicin, amikacin, neomycin and framycetin); the tetracyclines (tetracycline, chlortetracycline – aureomycin, methacycline, oxytetracycline – terramycin and others); and the imidazoles (metronidazole – flagyl, ketoconazole, miconazole, nimorazole, mebendazole and thiabendazole). In addition to these, there are other individual antibiotics such as chloramphenicol, erythromycin, lincomycin, clindamycin and spectinomycin.

[S] *Powerful antibiotics often produce undesirable side-effects.*

[S] *Allergies to some, especially penicillin, are common and may be serious or even fatal.*

[S] *The aminoglycoside antibiotics, which include streptomycin and gentamycin, can cause deafness, permanent singing in the ears (tinnitus), kidney damage or interference with normal blood production if used in large dosage or in people who cannot excrete them normally.*

[S] *The tetracycline antibiotics, such as aureomycin and terramycin, can cause permanent staining of teeth if given to young children.*

[S] *Wide-spectrum antibiotics can destroy normal,*

health-giving body bacteria and allow over-growth of undesirable organisms such as the candida fungus that causes thrush.

[S] Most antibiotic drugs can cause nausea and intestinal upset, diarrhoea and skin rashes.

Ideally, antibiotics should be used only for serious, or potentially serious infections or to prevent dangerous conditions in specially susceptible people. When a course is prescribed, it should be taken completely and the dosage should be regular.

anticancer drugs

drugs used to treat cancer. Most anticancer drugs are cytotoxic drugs – drugs which destroy rapidly growing cells, but some are derivatives from, or synthetic analogues of, the sex hormones. Some cancers are 'hormone dependent', being stimulated in their growth by certain hormones. Thus, some kinds of breast cancer are stimulated to grow by oestrogens and can be discouraged by male sex hormones or by the drug tamoxifen which has anti-

---

KEY

The symbol **[O]** indicates that the drug is either available over-the-counter or that an over-the-counter drug with the same active ingredient or ingredients is available.

The symbol **[»]** indicates the forms in which the drug can be taken.

The symbol **[S]** sets out side-effects.

The symbol **[W]** indicates a drug recently withdrawn. These drugs should not be used.

---

oestrogenic properties. Paradoxically, the growth of some breast cancers, especially in elderly women, is discouraged by oestrogen hormones given in very high doses. Cancer of the prostate gland is male hormone dependent and can often be greatly diminished by treatment with a female sex hormone such as stilboestrol.

anticholinergic drugs
drugs that oppose the action of the neuro-

transmitter acetylcholine in the body. Acetylcholine is released at many nerve endings in the parasympathetic part of the autonomic nervous system. These connections are responsible for the contraction of certain involuntary muscles, such as those of the iris of the eye and the bladder, the production of saliva, respiratory secretions and sweat, slowing the heart and increasing the activity of the bowels.

[S] *Anticholinergic drugs block the receptors for acetylcholine and the result is a dry mouth, a dry, hot skin, dilated pupils, a rapid heartbeat, relief of bowel colic and difficulty in emptying the bladder.*

The archetypal anticholinergic drug is belladonna (ATROPINE).

Such 'atropine-like' drugs are useful in drying up secretions prior to an operation, in the treatment of an unduly slow heart rate, the irritable bowel syndrome and certain types of urinary incontinence. They are used to treat Parkinson's disease, asthma, and motion sickness.

[S] *Overdosage, in addition to the effects mentioned, also causes difficulty in swallowing, retention of urine, blurred vision, anxiety, delirium, hallucinations, confusion and convulsions.*

Other anticholinergic drugs are hyoscine, scopolamine, homatropine, banthine, propantheline and dibutoline.

anticoagulant drugs
drugs which reduce the normal tendency of blood to clot and which are able to prevent clots forming in the circulation and to prevent the extension of existing clots. Anticoagulants work better in the veins than in the arteries and are most useful in the prevention and treatment of deep vein thrombosis. They are important in the prevention of clot formation on artificial heart valves or when an artificial kidney (dialysis machine) is in use.

Anticoagulants have no effect on clots which have already formed. Existing clots can only be dissolved by thrombolytic drugs. Nevertheless, these drugs are of value in reducing the likelihood of thrombosis or embolism and thus preventing stroke and other serious conditions.

The most important anticoagulant drug is the body's own natural anticoagulant, HEPARIN. This is still the most generally useful drug. Heparin blocks the activity of various coagulation factors needed for the clotting of the blood. It must be given by injection at least every six hours and it begins to work within a few hours.

Other anticoagulant drugs may be taken by mouth but are slow to take effect. Often these are started along with heparin, and the heparin injections stopped after three days. Oral anticoagulants include warfarin, nicoumalone, phenindione and the antiplatelet drugs protamine sulphate, dipyridamole and sulphinpyrazone.

Anticoagulant drugs must be used with great care and with constant monitoring of the blood clotting tendency to avoid the risk of severe haemorrhage.

anticonvulsant drugs
drugs used to prevent epileptic seizures and taken
continuously for long periods, usually twice a day.
A single drug, rather than a combination, is usually
preferred and the dose given is the least which
achieves the objective. A second drug may have to
be added if one fails to prevent attacks.
Anticonvulsant drugs are used in cases of
established epilepsy, in certain cases of head injury
in which there is a tendency to seizures, in the
emergency treatment of a prolonged seizure and
sometimes to prevent seizures in children with a
history of fits during fevers (febrile seizures).

The choice of drug depends on the type of seizure
and on the person's response. Most cases of
epilepsy can be well controlled with one or other
of the commonly used drugs – Epanutin
(phenytoin), primidone, tegretol (Carbamazepine),
phenobarbitone, sodium valproate, ethosuximide
or clonazepam.

antidepressant drugs

drugs used to treat depression. Three main groups of drugs are used – the tricyclics, the monoamine-oxidase (MAO) inhibitors and the SELECTIVE SEROTONIN RE-UPTAKE INHIBITOR DRUGS. The tricyclics and the serotonin re-uptake inhibitors are generally preferred because they are more effective and do not react dangerously, as the MAO inhibitors can, with certain foodstuffs and drugs. Other drugs used in the treatment of depression include lithium, flupenthixol, tryptophan and trazodone.

Among the most important tricyclic antidepressants are Tryptizole (amitriptyline), Tofranil (imipramine), Sinequan (doxepin), Anafranil (clomipramine) and Aventyl (nortriptyline). These drugs do not act quickly and it is important for the person taking them to understand that up to three weeks may be needed for the full effect to be achieved. They are usually taken for at least three months and may be followed by a long period on reduced dosage.

There are many different neuro-transmitters in the

body, but the most important are substances, similar to adrenaline, called monoamines. There is reason to believe that depression is caused by a shortage, or decreased effectiveness, of these substances at the nerve endings. Too much monoamine and we get overactivity, elation, an exaggerated sense of well-being, even mania. Not enough, and we get black depression.

Most antidepressant drugs can cause atropine-like effects such as dryness of the mouth, blurring of vision, constipation, difficulty in urination and drowsiness. Overdosage can be dangerous, even fatal.

MAO inhibitors, while valuable, are, however, potentially dangerous and people taking them must on no account eat cheese, pickled herring or broad bean pods, or eat or drink Marmite, Oxo, Bovril or any similar meat or yeast extract, Chianti wine, alcohol, except in moderation, or any medicines of any kind without the knowledge and consent of the doctor. The MAO inhibitor drugs act by blocking the action of enzymes which normally break down amine neuro-transmitters, thus allowing these to accumulate and stimulate brain action. But they also have the same effect on various amine drugs and food constituents, such as tyramine, and the active ingredients of these may accumulate in the body, causing a dangerous rise in blood pressure with severe headache. MAO inhibitors are marketed under names such as Marplan, Marsilid, Nardil and Parnate.

antidiabetic drugs
drugs used to treat Type I (insulin-dependent) or Type II (maturity onset) diabetes. Insulin is the body's sugar-regulating hormone and is produced by the pancreas and released into the blood in quantities which depend on the amount of sugar in the blood passing through the pancreas. Insulin controls the passage of sugar through the walls of muscle and fat cells and promotes the storage of sugar in the liver. Without it, muscles waste and the amounts of sugar and toxic acids in the blood rise to a high and dangerous level. Insulin-dependent diabetics are people who are able to produce little or no insulin for themselves and require to take it,

by injection, once, twice or sometimes three times a day.

Insulin can be obtained from pigs and oxen. These insulins differ slightly from human insulin, and unmodified insulin can stimulate the production of anti-insulin antibodies. Pig insulin can be modified to be identical to human insulin, but the latter is now extensively produced by recombinant DNA methods (genetic engineering). It has been widely claimed that human insulin used by diabetics does not give the same warning of hypoglycaemia as former insulins. This has been disputed by many experts.

Insulin solutions are now usually made in a strength of 100 units per millilitre, and syringes are calibrated in these units. Pure insulin acts rapidly and for a short time. Insulin zinc suspensions are released more slowly than 'soluble insulin' and their effect lasts longer. Various preparations, of varying duration of action, are used, often mixed with soluble insulin, as in the preparations Mixtard and Initard. Isophane insulin is an insulin of intermediate duration of action. Long duration 'slow' insulins include Ultralente, Semilente, and PZI (protamine zinc insulin).

People who can produce some insulin, but not enough, are said to have Type II, or maturity-onset, diabetes. If they are overweight, reducing may suffice, but often they require drugs which stimulate the pancreas to release stored insulin. For this to be successful, about one third of the insulin-producing tissue must still be functional. Given to normal people, drugs for Type II diabetes cause a severe drop in the blood sugar level (hypoglycaemia).

Commonly used hypoglycaemic drugs include Rastinon (tolbutamide), Diabinese (chlorpropamide), Daonil (glibenclamide) and Glucophage (metformin).

antidiarrhoeal drugs
drugs used to check diarrhoea. These may either be narcotics like codeine, which reduce the irritability of the bowel wall and cut down the rate of

contraction of the bowel muscles, or substances, such as methyl cellulose or a high fibre diet, which increase the bulk and solidity of the bowel contents. Other substances, such as chalk, ispaghula husk or kaolin, can be useful. Narcotic preparations include codeine, Lomotil (diphenoxylate), Imodium (loperamide), kaolin and morphine mixture, and aromatic chalk and opium.

Diarrhoea often serves to dispose of an irritant, such as infecting organisms, and should not be immediately checked. But diarrhoea persisting for more than two days is usually treated.

antidote
a drug which neutralizes or counteracts the action or effect of a poison. There are few specific antidotes. These include NALOXONE for narcotic opiate poisoning, desferrioxamine for iron poisoning, cobalt edetate for cyanide poisoning and n-acetylcysteine for paracetamol poisoning. Activated charcoal may be valuable to adsorb poisons.

```
KEY
The symbol [O] indicates that the drug is either
available over-the-counter or that an over-the-
counter drug with the same active ingredient or
ingredients is available.

The symbol [»] indicates the forms in which the
drug can be taken.

The symbol [S] sets out side-effects.

The symbol [W] indicates a drug recently
withdrawn. These drugs should not be used.
```

anti-emetic drugs

drugs used to relieve nausea and prevent vomiting
from whatever cause. They are useful in the control
of motion sickness, the nausea associated with
various kinds of vertigo including the vertigo of
Ménière's disease and the nausea associated with
medical treatment with powerful and toxic drugs
or sometimes with radiotherapy. They are valuable
in the management of the nausea and vomiting
associated with the effects of kidney failure

(uraemia), widespread cancer, radiation sickness, and acute gastro-enteritis caused by viruses. Sometimes, if the vomiting is severe, the drugs may have to be given rectally or by injection.

It is, in general, wrong to use anti-emetic drugs to treat nausea and vomiting caused by a disease, when an effective remedy exists for the cause, or to use them when the cause of the vomiting is unknown. To do so may be to conceal the cause and prevent definitive treatment. They are seldom used in diseases of the intestines, for instance.

ANTIHISTAMINE drugs, such as cyclizine, and anticholinergic drugs, such as hyoscine, can act as anti-emetics by dampening down nerve impulses from the balancing mechanisms in the inner ears. Other anti-emetics include atropine, Largactil (chlorpromazine), Stemetil (prochlorperazine), Fentazin (perphenazine) and Stelazine (trifluoperazine).

antifungal drugs
a group of drugs which act directly on the cell walls

of the various fungi which affect the skin and, less commonly, the internal organs. Antifungal drugs may be applied directly to the skin or mucous membranes in the form of creams, lotions, solutions or powders, or may be taken by mouth. For very severe internal fungal infections antifungal drugs may have to be given by injection.

Antifungal drugs are used in the treatment of the various kinds of tinea, in the control of thrush (candidiasis), whether of the skin, the vagina, the mouth or the internal organs, and in the management of a number of rare internal fungus infections, such as cryptococcosis or torulopsis.

Major antifungal drugs, for internal use, include Fungilin (amphotericin), Alcobon (flucytosine) and griseofulvin. Local applications include Canesten (clotrimazole) [0], miconazole, econazole and Nystan (nystatin).

antihistamine drugs
drugs that oppose the action of histamine in the body by blocking the receptors for histamine on

cells. Histamine is a powerful agent produced in
the body by certain cells called mast cells, especially
as an allergic response. It acts on small blood
vessels, causing them to widen and to become
abnormally permeable to protein molecules so that
these escape into the tissue fluid and cause
oedema. The antihistamine group of drugs act
against histamine and are thus useful in the
treatment of many allergic conditions including hay
fever (allergic rhinitis), asthma, urticaria, and other
allergic rashes. They are commonly incorporated
into cold and cough 'remedies' because of their
symptomatic effect and are valuable in the
suppression of vomiting.

[S] *Side-effects are common with antihistamine
drugs and include sedation, sleepiness, loss of
coordination, blurred vision, dizziness, loss of
appetite, nausea, dry mouth and difficulty in
passing urine.*

The list of antihistamines is long but among the
most important are acrivastine (Semprex),
antazoline (Antistin-Privine), astemizole (Hismanal),

azatadine (Optimine), azelastine (Rhinolast), brompheniramine (Dimotane Plus), chlorpheniramine (Aller-chlor, Haymine, Piriton, Phenetron), clemastine (Tavegil), cyproheptadine (Periactin), dimethindine maleate (Vibrocil), hydroxyzine hydrochloride (Atarax), ketotifen (Zaditen), loratadine (Clarityn), mequitazine (Primalan), oxatomide (Tinset), phenindamine (Thephorin), pheniramine (Daneral), promethazine (Phenergan), terfenadine (Triludan), trimeprazine (Vallergan) and triprolidine (Actidil, Actifed, Pro-Actidil).

antihypertensive drugs

drugs used for the control of abnormally raised blood pressure (hypertension) so as to prevent complications such as stroke, heart attack (myocardial infarction), heart failure and kidney damage. Unfortunately, high blood pressure produces obvious symptoms only when it is severe or has already reached a fairly advanced stage and has caused damage to the blood vessels and the heart. So it has to be looked for. Every adult should have regular checks. Proper and effective treatment can largely eliminate the additional risk of these serious complications.

Three main classes of drugs are used to treat high blood pressure. The first, the diuretics, act on the kidneys to cause them to pass more water and salt in the urine and reduce the volume of the blood, so bringing down the pressure. The second group, the beta-blockers, interfere with the hormone and nervous control of the heart, slowing it and causing it to beat less forcefully, so reducing the pressure. The third group, the vasodilators, act on the arteries to widen them. This group contains drugs acting in quite different ways. They include the alpha blockers, the calcium channel blockers and the ACE inhibitors.

The treatment of high blood pressure is not simply a matter of prescribing tablets. The doctor has difficult and complex decisions to make. Among others, he or she has to decide whether to use drugs at all. Because the body may have adapted to raised blood pressure, reducing it may actually cause the person concerned to feel worse, rather than better. Until the body readjusts to normal pressures, there may be a sense of weakness and loss of energy, depression and a tendency to dizziness or faintness on standing up. The doctor aims to achieve control with the minimum dosage and will want to monitor the pressure regularly.

Many other factors besides drugs are important in the treatment of high blood pressure. These include weight control, exercise and the avoidance of smoking.

anti-inflammatory drugs
drugs that prevent or reverse the redness, heat, pain, swelling and loss of function which are the characteristics of inflammation. They include the non-steroidal anti-inflammatory drugs and the CORTICOSTEROID DRUGS.

antimalarial
a drug used to treat or prevent malaria.

antimetabolite
an anticancer, or cytotoxic, drug which acts by

143

combining with essential enzymes within cancer cells so as to interfere with their growth. To be useful, antimetabolites must be significantly more toxic to cancer cells than to normal cells.

antimetabolites
anticancer drugs.

antimicrobial
able to destroy microorganisms. See ANTIBIOTIC DRUGS.

antimitotic
an anticancer drug, or agency, which acts by interfering with the reproduction of cancer cells.

antimitotic drugs
drugs that interfere with the reproduction and growth of cells and are used as anticancer drugs.

antimonials
antimony-containing drugs, especially the pentavalent group such as sodium stibogluconate (stibophen) and meglumine antimoniate, used in

the treatment of kala-azar (leishmaniasis).

antimycotic
a drug used in the treatment of fungus infections.

antimycotic drugs
ANTIFUNGAL DRUGS.

antineoplastic
able to control the growth or spread of cancers
(neoplasms).

anti-oestrogen drug
one of a group of drugs that oppose the action of
the female sex hormone oestrogen. The most
important of these drugs is tamoxifen, which
antagonizes the action of oestrogens at the tissue
receptors. Anti-oestrogen drugs are used to assist in
the treatment of breast cancer and to stimulate
egg production (ovulation) in infertile women.

[S] *Side-effects include hot flushes, itching of the*
vulva, nausea, vomiting, fluid retention and
sometimes vaginal bleeding.

145

KEY

The symbol **[0]** indicates that the drug is either available over-the-counter or that an over-the-counter drug with the same active ingredient or ingredients is available.

The symbol **[»]** indicates the forms in which the drug can be taken.

The symbol **[S]** sets out side-effects.

The symbol **[W]** indicates a drug recently withdrawn. These drugs should not be used.

---

anti-oxidants

substances capable of neutralizing oxygen free radicals, the highly active and damaging atoms and chemical groups produced by various disease processes and by poisons, radiation, smoking and other agencies. The body contains its own natural anti-oxidants but there is growing medical interest in the possibility of controlling cell and tissue damage by means of supplementary anti-oxidants. Those most commonly used are vitamin C (ascorbic acid) and vitamin E (tocopherols). Evidence is accumulating that these substances, in adequate dosage, can reduce the incidence of a number of serious diseases.

antiparkinsonism drugs
drugs used to control the effects of Parkinson's disease. They include levodopa (Sinemet), amantadine (Symmetrel), bromocriptine (Parlodel) and selegiline (Eldepryl).

antiperspirants
substances used to reduce the rate of sweating in certain areas of the body where the sweat glands produce sweat that is especially likely to cause body odour. These are called apocrine glands and occur mainly in the armpits (axillae) and groins. The sweat from the apocrine glands is broken down by bacteria to form odorous substances.

Antiperspirants have an astringent action, narrowing or obstructing the outlet of the sweat glands. Used in excess they may cause skin irritation. They are often combined with

deodorants. (see DEODORISING DRUGS). Common
antiperspirants are alum, aluminium chloride and
aluminium chlorohydrate.

antipruritics

any substance which relieves itching. Calamine
lotions or creams are safe and popular, but
sometimes more powerful remedies are required,
such as local anaesthetics or local ANTIHISTAMINES.
Both of these are liable to cause skin sensitisation
and are not much approved of by dermatologists.

Antihistamines are sometimes given by mouth for
itching. Eurax (crotamiton) is often prescribed.

antipsychotic drugs

drugs used to treat the major mental illnesses such
as the various forms of schizophrenia, manic
depressive illness, mania and major depression.
Antipsychotic drugs are also used to control the
behaviour of people who are seriously agitated or
aggressive. The drug treatment of psychosis has
revolutionized psychiatry and has greatly reduced
the number of people confined in mental hospitals

The most commonly used antipsychotic drugs are the phenothiazine derivatives such as Largactil (chlorpromazine), Depixol (flupenthixol), Orap (pimozide), Melleril (thioridazine) and Sparine (promazine). Lithium is valuable in the management of mania and manic-depressive illness. Most of these drugs act by blocking the action of the neuro-transmitter dopamine. Lithium is believed to cut down the production of another neuro-transmitter, norepinephrine.

[S] *These powerful drugs have side-effects, some of which are distressing. Most of them can cause regular jerky movements of some part of the body (dyskinesia) or parkinsonism – a disorder with effects similar to those of Parkinson's disease – and lethargy and drowsiness are common.*

[S] *Other side-effects include dryness of the mouth, blurred vision and difficulty in passing urine.*

[S] *Lithium must be given in very carefully regulated dosage, and toxic effects are common.*

149

These include tremor, staggering (ataxia), jerking of the eyes (nystagmus), difficulty in speaking and seizures.

antipyretic drugs

drugs which lower raised body temperature. In fever, the body's thermostat is temporarily set at a higher then normal level, so one feels cold and shivering occurs to increase body heat to the required level. Antipyretic drugs reset the thermostat to a normal level. The use of drugs for this purpose is less popular than it was prior to the introduction of ANTIBIOTICS. Nowadays more attention is devoted to removing the cause of the fever – usually infection. The commonest antipyretic drug is aspirin (acetylsalicylic acid) or paracetamol for children.

antirabies serum

serum containing specific antibodies against rabies, used to prevent the development of the disease in those who have been bitten by a rabid animal.

antirachitic
acting against rickets or the development of
rickets.

antirheumatic
any treatment for, or prophylaxis against, any form
of rheumatism.

antirheumatic drugs
drugs used to treat any form of rheumatism,
especially rheumatoid arthritis and osteoarthritis.
Rheumatoid arthritis and associated conditions are
caused by a disorder of the body's immune system
which leads it to attacks its own tissues.

The most powerful antirheumatic drugs operate by
interfering with the functioning of the immune
system and these include the CORTICOSTEROID
DRUGS and other immunosuppressive drugs.
Rheumatoid arthritis is often treated with
penicillamine (not to be confused with the
ANTIBIOTIC drug penicillin), gold,
hydroxychloroquine and chloroquine.

The non-steroidal anti-inflammatory drugs are commonly used. Drugs such as paracetamol and the narcotic ANALGESIC drugs may be useful in relieving pain, but have no anti-inflammatory action.

All the major antirheumatic drugs may produce serious side-effects. Penicillamine and gold can damage the kidneys, chloroquine can destroy the unction of the central part of the retinas causing severe loss of vision, and CORTICOSTEROID DRUGS may cause osteoporosis, may reactivate latent infections or reduce resistance to new infections, and may lead to severe shock in the event of injury or other major illness.

antiscorbutic
tending to prevent, or able to cure, scurvy. The antiscorbutic substance is vitamin C (ascorbic acid).

antiseptics
mildly antibacterial substances, usually applied to the skin in the form of solutions, to try to reduce the chance of infection. They are of limited value

and do not reduce the importance of thorough washing and cleansing. Alcohol, iodine, pHisohex (hexachlorophane), Cetavlon (cetrimide) **[O]**, Alphosyl (allantoin and coal tar), benzalkonium, Thimerosal (thiomersal) and hydrogen peroxide are among the many substances used as skin antiseptics.

antiserum

animal or human blood serum, which contains useful immunoglobulins (antibodies) to organisms with which the animal has been deliberately infected or to the toxins produced by these organisms (antitoxins).

Such serum can be life-saving but can also cause severe reactions. It is usually given by injection into a muscle, and the danger of a severe allergic reaction (anaphylactic shock) is ever present in the mind of the doctor, who will first give a very small test dose just under the skin.

Sera are used for the treatment of conditions such as diphtheria, tetanus, rabies, chicken-pox and shingles, and Lassa fever.

A range of different antisera is used in medical laboratories to identify unknown organisms. Visible clumping of the organisms will occur when the right serum is added.

AntiSpas
a trade name for BENZHEXOL.

antispasmodic drugs
drugs which relax tight contraction (spasm) in involuntary (smooth) muscle in any part of the body, but especially in the wall of the intestine or the bladder. These drugs act by blocking the action of the neuro-transmitter acetylcholine, which is released from the nerve endings that stimulate the muscle contraction. They are useful in the treatment of bowel colic, as in the irritable bowel syndrome, and in bladder spasm in cystitis and other conditions. Antispasmodic drugs are anticholinergic drugs.

anti-tetanus serum
a serum containing specific antibodies against
TETANUS, usually obtained from a horse which has
been inoculated with tetanus organisms and has
developed immunity to the disease. People who
have had tetanus toxoid immunization are spared
the possible allergic dangers of anti-tetanus serum.

antitussive
a drug used to relieve or abolish coughing.

antivenin
one of a range of specific antidotes for the bites of
venomous animals such as snakes, centipedes,
spiders and scorpions. Antivenins are held by
doctors in areas in which venomous bites are
common and identification of the animal
concerned is important. They are prepared by
injecting small and increasing doses of the venom
into animals such as horses so that antibodies will
be produced with specific action against the
venom. Such antibodies neutralize the venoms and
are called antivenins.

antivenom
see ANTIVENIN.

antiviral drugs
drugs effective against viruses that cause disease. For many years after the introduction of the ANTIBIOTICS it seemed unlikely that a comparable group of drugs with action against viruses would ever be developed.

Viruses are fundamentally different from bacteria and larger organisms in that they can only reproduce and survive within living cells. It is thus very difficult to find a drug capable of destroying viruses which is not also liable to destroy the host cell.

There have been no fundamental breakthroughs in antiviral therapy, but a number of small advances based on advances in knowledge of the biochemistry and nuclear biology of viruses.

The most successful approaches, to date, have exploited ways of interfering with the replication

KEY

The symbol [O] indicates that the drug is either available over-the-counter or that an over-the-counter drug with the same active ingredient or ingredients is available.

The symbol [»] indicates the forms in which the drug can be taken.

The symbol [S] sets out side-effects.

The symbol [W] indicates a drug recently withdrawn. These drugs should not be used.

of virus DNA or RNA either by blocking the enzymes which promote this process (the polymerases) or by inserting new instructions into the DNA to order a stop to the process (chain-terminators). Early drugs, acting on these principles were Herplex (idoxuridine), Trifluridine, Vidarabine and Acyclovir. These drugs are all active against the herpes viruses and the latter, in particular, has had a great success. It is, at the time of writing, the most useful antiviral drug available and has saved many lives in immunocompromised people with widespread herpes infections, as well as preventing an immense amount of pain and distress in people with genital herpes infections and shingles.

The success of acyclovir has encouraged the development of similar drugs such as DHPG (GANCICLOVIR) which is more active against the human cytomegalovirus, and AZT (zidovudine) which has some useful action in suppressing the replication of the AIDS virus HIV.

[S] *Unfortunately, AZT is toxic and affects blood production in the bone marrow.*

Some viruses make use of an enzyme, reverse transcriptase, to promote the production of the replicated half of the double helix. This enzyme has been closely studied by workers hoping to be able to block its action, because any drug capable of doing this would stop the reproduction of the virus concerned. The substances dideoxycytidine and Foscarnet (phosphonoformate) are able to do this. Foscarnet can also inhibit the polymerases of all herpes viruses, but it too is toxic.

Ribavirin, acting in a different way, interferes with the replication of a range of viruses including many dangerous respiratory viruses for which effective drugs are badly needed. Some experimental success has been achieved, using the drug in aerosols, against some influenza strains and in serious respiratory syncytial virus infections in children and in Lassa fever. Amantadine and Rimantadine are useful against Influenza A virus.

Interferons are substances produced by cells as part of the natural defence against virus infections. The do not act directly against viruses but modify other cells so that they become less capable of cooperating with viruses in achieving the assembly of their components and their replication. Genetic engineering techniques (recombinant DNA) have enabled us to produce enough interferons for clinical trials and some limited clinical use, and results are encouraging. The common cold can be treated by direct application to the nose lining, but there are side-effects and the treatment is

159

uneconomically expensive. Genital warts and hepatitis B have been successfully treated.

We are only at the beginning of a process which, if current expectations are realised, may parallel the remarkable advances achieved in the development of the ANTIBIOTICS in the last fifty years.

Antraderm
a trade name for DITHRANOL.

anxiolytic
a drug used to treat anxiety.

aperient
a laxative or mild purgative.

aphrodisiac
a drug purporting to stimulate sexual interest or excitement or enhance sexual performance.

Apresoline
a trade name for HYDRALAZINE.

Aprinox

a trade name for BENDROFLUAZIDE.

aprotinin

a drug that prevents the breakdown of blood clots and helps to control bleeding.

[»] *An antifibrinolytic drug administered by injection.*

A trade name is Trasylol.

ara-A

adenine arabinoside or vidarabine. This is an analogue of the deoxyribonucleoside of adenine and acts by inhibiting DNA polymerase. It is effective against herpes viruses, varicella-zoster virus, vaccinia and hepatitis B viruses.

Arpimycin

a trade name for erythromycin, an ANTIBIOTIC.

arsphenamine

an organic arsenical compound formerly used to

treat syphilis. Treatment with arsenical drugs was called arsenotherapy.

Artane
a trade name for BENZHEXOL.

Artracin
a trade name for INDOMETHACIN.

Ascabiol
a trade name for BENZYL BENZOATE.

Ascalix
a trade name for PIPERAZINE.

ascorbic acid
vitamin C. A white, crystalline substance found in citrus fruits, tomatoes, potatoes, and leafy green vegetables. Small doses are needed to prevent the bleeding disease of scurvy and large doses are believed to be useful in combatting dangerous free radicals.

Asilone
a trade name for ALUMINIUM HYDROXIDE. [O]

Asmaven
a trade name for SALBUTAMOL.

aspartame
an artificial sweetener derived from aspartic acid and phenylalanine.

aspirin
acetylsalicylic acid. A drug used as a pain-killer, to reduce fever, or as a means of reducing the tendency of blood to clot within the circulation. Aspirin is a prostaglandin inhibitor and this accounts for the wide range of its actions. [O]

Aspro
a trade name for ASPIRIN. [O]

Asprodeine
a trade name for ASPIRIN and CODEINE. [O]

astemizole
an ANTIHISTAMINE drug used to treat hay fever and allergic skin conditions.

[S] *Side-effects include weight gain and, on very high dosage, heart irregularity.*

A trade name is Hismanal.

astringent
a drug that shrinks cells and tightens surfaces by denaturing cell protein.

Atarax
a trade name for HYDROXYZINE.

atenolol
a beta adrenoceptor blocker drug that acts mostly on the heart and has a long action. It slows the heart and corrects irregularities of rhythm. A trade name is Tenormin.

Atensine
a trade name for DIAZEPAM.

Ativan
a trade name for LORAZEPAM.

atracurium besylate
a drug used by anaesthetists that causes profound muscle relaxation. A trade name is Tracrium.

Atromid-S
a trade name for CLOFIBRATE.

atropine
a bitter, poisonous alkaloid obtained from the plant Atropa belladonna ('deadly nightshade') and the seeds of the Thorn-apple. It blocks acetyl choline receptors and is used to relax spasm in smooth muscle in the intestines and other organs. It is also extensively used by ophthalmologists to dilate the pupil of the eye in the treatment of inflammatory disease and sometimes to facilitate examination. The generic term derives from the Greek a, not, and tropos, turning. Atropos was one of the three fates noted for her inexorable tendency to cut the thread of life.

KEY

The symbol **[O]** indicates that the drug is either available over-the-counter or that an over-the-counter drug with the same active ingredient or ingredients is available.

The symbol **[»]** indicates the forms in which the drug can be taken.

The symbol **[S]** sets out side-effects.

The symbol **[W]** indicates a drug recently withdrawn. These drugs should not be used.

---

auranofin

a gold preparation used to treat rheumatoid arthritis.

[S] *Side-effects include nausea, abdominal pain, diarrhoea and mouth ulcers. A trade name is Ridaura.*

Aureomycin

a trade name for the ANTIBIOTIC
CHLORTETRACYCLINE.

Austramycin

a trade name for TETRACYCLINE.

Austrapen

a trade name for AMPICILLIN.

Avil

a trade name for PHENIRAMINE.

Avloclor

a trade name for CHLOROQUINE.

Avomine

a trade name for PROMETHAZINE.

Azactam

a trade name for AZTREONAM.

Azamune

a trade name for AZATHIOPRINE.

azapropazone
an NSAID used to treat rheumatoid arthritis, osteoarthritis, ankylosing spondylitis and gout. A trade name is Rheumox.

azatadine
an ANTIHISTAMINE and serotonin antagonist drug use to treat hat fever, urticaria, itching and stings. A trade name is Optimine.

azathioprine
a drug used to suppress the immune system so as to avoid rejection of donor transplants.

[S] *Immune suppression may have serious side-effects such as the flare-up of latent infections and an increased risk of malignant tumours such as lymphomas, but azathioprine is safer than other immunosuppressive drugs.*

Azathioprine is also used to treat rheumatism. A trade name is Imuran.

azelaic acid
an antibacterial drug administered as a cream for external application in the treatment of acne. A trade name is Skinoren.

azelastine
an ANTIHISTAMINE drug administered as a metered-dose nasal spray for the treatment of hay fever. A trade name is Rhinolast.

Azide
a trade name for CHLOROTHIAZIDE.

azithromycin
an ANTIBIOTIC drug used to treat respiratory, skin, soft tissue and other infections, especially those caused by the organism Chlamydia trachomatis. A trade name is Zithromax.

azlocillin
an ANTIBIOTIC drug, administered by intravenous infusion, to treat infections especially those caused by the dangerous organism Pseudomonas aeruginosa. A trade name is Securopen.

AZT
abbreviation for azidothymidine or Zidovudine. A drug used in attempts to control AIDS.

[S] *The drug is toxic but does seem to be able to prolong life.*

aztreonam
an ANTIBIOTIC drug used to treat infections of the lungs, bones, skin and soft tissues with organisms of the Gram stain negative class (Gram-negative organisms). It is especially useful in lung infections in children with cystic fibrosis. A trade name is Azactam.

bacampicillin
a semisynthetic penicillin ANTIBIOTIC. It is a derivative of ampicillin with improved absorption, giving higher blood levels than the parent substance.

bacitracin
an ANTIBIOTIC derived from the bacterium Bacillus subtilis. It acts by interfering with the formation of

the bacterial cell membrane and is highly effective against many organisms especially the haemolytic streptococcus.

Unfortunately, it is so liable to damage the kidneys that it must be confined to external use.

baclofen

a drug derived from the neuro-transmitter GABA that interferes with nerve transmission in the spinal cord and relaxes muscle spasm. It is used to alleviate the effects of conditions such as stroke and multiple sclerosis. A trade name is Lioresal.

Bactrim

a trade name for CO-TRIMOXAZOLE.

Banocide

a trade name for DIETHYLCARBAMAZINE.

Baratol

a trade name for INDORAMIN.

barbiturates drugs

a range of sedative drugs derived from barbituric acid. The barbiturates were formerly used in enormous quantities, but are now largely replaced by the BENZODIAZAPINE DRUGS The best known barbiturates are Luminal (phenobarbitone), Amytal (amylobarbitone) Soneryl (butobarbitone) and Pentothal (thiopentone). Apart from phenobarbitone for epilepsy and pentothal for the induction of general anaesthesia, they are now largely out of fashion and are beginning to acquire the same disreputable air, in medical circles, as the once equally highly regarded amphetamines. Much the same thing is now beginning to happen to the benzodiazepines.

The origin of the term 'barbiturate' is on a par with the name of the benzodiazepine 'Mogadon' (which is said to have been tested on moggies). Johann Friedrich Wilhelm Baeyer, the Nobel prize winner, who was working on new derivatives of urea, a constituent of urine, is claimed to have obtained the supplies of urea from which he synthesized the new compound, from a Munich waitress called

Barbara. So Barbara's uric acid became barbituric acid.

Barbloc
a trade name for PINDOLOL.

Barbopent
a trade name for PENTOBARBITONE.

Becloforte
a trade name for BECLOMETHASONE.

beclomethasone
a CORTICOSTEROID DRUG used in the form of a nasal spray to relieve the symptoms of hay fever (allergic rhinitis). It is also used to treat asthma. Trade names are Beconase and Becotide.

Beconase
a trade name for BECLOMETHASONE.

Becotide
a trade name for BECLOMETHASONE.

belladonna
a crude form of ATROPINE derived from the leaves
and roots of the poisonous plant, Atropa
belladonna. The term derives from the cosmetic use
of the alkaloid to widen the pupils. Bella donna is
Italian for beautiful woman.

Benadon
a trade name for PYRIDOXINE.

Benadryl
a trade name for DIPHENHYDRAMINE. [0]

bendrofluazide
a thiazide DIURETIC drug used to treat high blood
pressure (hypertension) and heart failure. Trade
names are Aprinox, Centyl and Inderex.

Benemid
a trade name for PROBENECID.

benorylate
a drug derived from ASPIRIN and PARACETAMOL
which is less irritating to the stomach than aspirin,

but equally effective as a pain-killer and non-steroidal anti-inflammatory drug. A trade name is Benoral.

Benoxyl
a trade name for BENZOYL PEROXIDE.

benperidol
a butyrophenone antipsychotic drug used to treat deviant sexual behaviour. A trade name is Anquil.

benserazide
a drug given in conjunction with levodopa to prevent its breakdown in the body. A trade name is Madopar.

Benylin
a trade name for DIPHENHYDRAMINE with other ingredients. [O]

Benyphed
a trade name for a mixture of DIPHENHYDRAMINE, DEXTROMETHORPHAN, PHENYLEPHRINE and other drugs. [O]

Benzac
a trade name for BENZOYL PEROXIDE.

Benzagel
a trade name for BENZOYL PEROXIDE.

benzalkonium
an antiseptic used in solution for skin and wound cleansing and as a means of sterilizing eye drops and contact lens solutions.

[S] *Allergic reactions occur.*

A trade name is Drapolene.

benzathine penicillin
an early, long-acting penicillin that must be given by injection.

Benzedrine
a trade name for AMPHETAMINE.

benzerazide
a dopamine precursor and dopa decarboxylase

KEY
The symbol **[O]** indicates that the drug is either available over-the-counter or that an over-the-counter drug with the same active ingredient or ingredients is available.

The symbol **[»]** indicates the forms in which the drug can be taken.

The symbol **[S]** sets out side-effects.

The symbol **[W]** indicates a drug recently withdrawn. These drugs should not be used.

inhibitor drug used to treat parkinsonism following encephalitis (post-encephalitic parkinsonism). A trade name is Madopar.

benzhexol
an anticholinergic drug that blocks the action of acetylcholine in the nervous system. It is used to treat the symptoms of Parkinson's disease.

benzocaine

a tasteless white powder with powerful local anesthetic properties.

[»] *Often used in lozenges in combination with antiseptics.*

A trade name is Tyrozets.

benzodiazepine drugs

a range of sedative and tranquillizing drugs of the Valium, Librium and Mogadon type. They were introduced in 1960 by Hoffman-LaRoche whose profits from this group alone have been astronomical. Compared with earlier sedatives, the benzodiazepines are remarkably safe and death from overdose is rare. They are prescribed and consumed by the billion, about 2 per cent of the population taking them regularly to promote sleep, reduce anxiety and relieve depression.

There is no question that they abolish much distress of mind. Equally there is no question that they do this more safely than the common alternative –

alcohol. It is surprising, however, that it is only recently that serious concern has been expressed over the inevitable dependence which must occur when one relies on a drug rather than on one's own resources. Dependence of this sort is not a property of any one particular drug, and the claim that any such drugs are not habit-forming is a semantic quibble.

In small doses the benzodiazepines relax muscles and relieve anxiety. In larger doses they put people to sleep. They include Mogadon (nitrazepam) and Dalmane (flurazepam) both of which have a prolonged action which may be cumulative; Halcion (triazolam) and Euhypnos (temazepam), which have a shorter action and no hangover effect; and Valium (diazepam), Librium (chlordiazepoxide), Ativan (lorazepam), Nobrium (medazepam) and Tranxene (clorazepate), all of which are widely used for the relief of mild anxiety.

benzopyrine
a yellow, crystalline, aromatic carcinogen found in coal tar and cigarette smoke.

benzoyl peroxide
a preparation used in the treatment of acne and
other skin conditions. It acts by removing the
surface layers of the epidermis and unblocking skin
pores, and has an antiseptic effect on skin bacteria.

[S] *Side-effects include skin irritation and*
excessive peeling, even, occasionally, blistering.

Trade names: Acetoxyl, Acnegel, Benoxyl.

benztropine
an anticholinergic drug used to control the
symptoms of Parkinson's disease.

benzydamine hydrochloride
an NSAID used to treat muscle pain. A trade name
is Difflam.

benzyl benzoate
an oily liquid used as a lotion for the treatment of scabies.

benzylpenicillin
the original highly active penicillin. The drug is destroyed by the digestive system and must be given by injection.

bephenium hydroxynaphthoate
an anthelmintic drug to get rid of hookworms and other nematodes. A trade name is Alcopar.

Berkatens
a trade name for VERAPAMIL.

Berkmycen
a trade name for OXYTETRACYCLINE.

Berocca
a trade name for a mixture of B vitamins and vitamin C.

Berotec
a trade name for FENOTEROL.

beta-blocker drugs
drugs that block the receptors on cells for
adrenaline-like natural substances. The term 'beta-
blocker' is an abbreviation of 'beta-adrenoreceptor
blocking agent'. The adrenoreceptors come in two
main classes, alpha and beta, and in several sub-
classes.

The beta receptors are sites on the heart, arteries,
muscles and elsewhere at which adrenaline and
related hormones act, in moments of stress and
need for action, to speed up the heart and constrict
blood vessels, so increasing the blood pressure,
reducing digestive processes and widening the
airway tubes in the lungs (bronchi).

The beta-blocker drugs chemically resemble
adrenaline and occupy these sites so that
adrenaline, although present, cannot act.

The result can be very advantageous for people

with angina, irregularities in the heartbeat, high
blood pressure (hypertension) and a tendency to
over-react to stress. But they can be very
disadvantageous to anyone with a tendency to
asthma, and can induce a severe asthmatic attack.

Many beta-blockers have been developed, some
with a greater action on one part of the body than
on another. Their generic names usually end in
'-olol'. The most commonly used beta-blockers
include Inderal (propranolol), Tenormin (atenolol),
Trandate (labetalol), Trasicor (oxprenolol) and
Sectral (acebutolol).

*One of the earliest beta-blockers, practolol, was
marketed in 1970 after the most stringent tests.
Four years later, after many thousands of patients
had used the drug, an alert eye specialist noted
that he was seeing patients with a most unusual
form of dry eye, in which the outer layer of the
cornea (the epithelium) was coming off in shreds.*

*All these patients were taking practolol and some
became blind. Soon it was found that the drug was*

also affecting the skin, the inner ear and the inner lining of the abdomen (the peritoneum). Only a small proportion of people on the drug were affected and some kind of immunological process was clearly involved.

The drug was withdrawn, except for special cases, and the manufacturer accepted moral responsibility and paid compensation. Beta-blockers in current use have no such effects.

Betadine
the trade name for POVIDONE IODINE, a mild antiseptic, which is used as a surgical scrub or as a lotion or ointment. [0]

Betadren
a trade name for PINDOLOL.

betahistine
a drug with properties similar to the natural body substance histamine, that is used to treat Ménière's disease. A common side-effect is nausea. A trade name is Serc.

beta-lactam antibiotics

a group of drugs that includes the penicillins and the cephalosporins. All have a 4 membered beta-lactam ring as part of the basic structure. Beta-lactam antibiotics function by interfering with the growth of a layer in the cell walls of bacteria that protects them from the environment. Without this layer the bacteria burst open and are destroyed.

Human cell walls do not have this layer; this is why these antibiotics are so safe. Bacteria protect themselves against these antibiotics by producing enzymes, beta-lactamases, that block this interference.

Betaloc

a trade name for metoprocol, a BETA-BLOCKER used to treat high blood pressure.

betamethasone

a CORTICOSTEROID DRUG used directly on the skin to treat eczema and psoriasis, by inhalation to treat asthma, by mouth for more severe allergic conditions and by injection to reduce brain swelling

KEY
The symbol **[O]** indicates that the drug is either available over-the-counter or that an over-the-counter drug with the same active ingredient or ingredients is available.

The symbol **[»]** indicates the forms in which the drug can be taken.

The symbol **[S]** sets out side-effects.

The symbol **[W]** indicates a drug recently withdrawn. These drugs should not be used.

in head injuries, tumour and infections. Trade names are Betnesol and Betnovate.

Betamin
a trade name for THIAMINE.

bethanechol
a cholinergic drug that acts mainly on the bowel and bladder, stimulating these organs to empty. A trade name is Kerlone, Betoptic.

Betim
a trade name for TIMOLOL.

Betnelan
a trade name for BETAMETHASONE.

Betnesol
a trade name for BETAMETHASONE.

Betnovate
a trade name for BETAMETHASONE.

bezafibrate
a cholesterol-lowering drug used to treat
abnormally high blood cholesterol levels
(hypercholesterolaemia) that fails to respond to
diet. A trade name is Bezalip.

Bezalip
a trade name for bezafibrate, a drug used to lower
blood cholesterol levels.

Bicillin
a trade name for benzathine PENICILLIN.

187

Bicnu
a trade name for carmustine, a CYTOTOXIC drug.

biguanides
drugs, such as METFORMIN and PHENFORMIN used to treat Type II diabetes. They are part of the group of oral hypoglycaemic drugs.

Biguanides act by reducing the efficiency of ION movement across cell membranes thus interfering with the production of glucose by the liver and reducing the energy yield from glucose used as fuel.

Biltricide
a trade name for PRAZIQUANTEL.

Biocitrin
a trade name for vitamin C.

Biogastrone [W]
a trade name for CARBENOXOLONE.

Biophylline [W]
a trade name for THEOPHYLLINE.

Bioplex
a trade name for CARBENOXOLONE.

Biorphen
a trade name for ORPHENADRINE.

Biotime
a trade name for a mixture of vitamins and minerals.

biotin
a water-soluble B vitamin concerned in the metabolism of fats and carbohydrates. Deficiency causes dermatitis, muscle pain, loss of appetite and anaemia.

Biovital
a trade name for a mixture of vitamins and minerals.

Biphasil

a trade name for an oral contraceptive.

Biquinate

a trade name for QUININE.

Bismag

a trade name for a mixture of baking soda (sodium bicarbonate) and magnesium carbonate.

bismuth

a drug used, as the carbonate, to treat peptic ulcer, especially when the organism Helicobacter pylori is a causal agent. Bismuth is also used, as the oxide or subgallate, for external use is soothing ointments. A trade name is (carbonate) APP, (oxide) Anusol.

bisoprolol

a beta-blocker drug used to treat angina pectoris. Trade names are Emcor and Monocor.

bithionol

a bacteriostatic agent useful against many organisms. It was formerly incorporated in medicated soaps. It is also used in the treatment of parasitic diseases such as paragonimiasis.

Blenoxane
a trade name for BLEOMYCIN.

bleomycin
a toxic glycopeptide ANTIBIOTIC that interferes with the synthesis of DNA and is used as an anticancer drug, usually in combination with other drugs. It has some value in Hodgkin's disease, other lymphomas and squamous cell cancers of the skin.

[S] *Side-effects include fibrosis of the lungs, drying and discoloration of the skin over the back of joints.*

Blocadren
a trade name for TIMOLOL.

borneol
an essential oil used, in conjunction with other essential oils, such as menthol, menthone and camphene, to disperse gallstones and kidney

stones. Trade names are Rowachol and Rowatinex.

botulinum toxin
a powerful nerve toxin produced by the organism
Clostridium botulinum which has been found to be
useful, in very small doses, in the treatment of an
increasing range of conditions such as squint
(strabismus) caused by overactive eye muscles or
uncontrollable spasm of the eyelid muscles. A trade
name is Dysport.

bretylium tosylate
a drug used in emergency to try to reverse the
rapidly fatal ventricular fibrillation, a form of
cardiac arrest, that has failed to respond to
attempts at electrical defibrillation. A trade name is
Bretylate.

Brevital
a short-acting barbiturate drug, methohexital
sodium, which is used as an induction agent during
general anaesthesia.

Bricanyl
a trade name for TERBUTALINE.

Brinaldix
a trade name for CLOPAMIDE.

Brocadopa
a trade name for levodopa, an immensely powerful ANTIPARKINSONISM drug.

Brolene
a trade name for an eye ointment containing DIBROMOPROPAMIDINE. [0]

bromazepam
a long-acting benzodiazepine drug used in the short-term treatment of disabling anxiety. A trade name is Loxetan.

bromocriptine
an ergot derivative drug with dopamine-like effects, used in the treatment of Parkinson's disease and to prevent lactation by inhibiting the secretion of the hormone prolactin by the pituitary gland.

[»]*The drug is administered by mouth.*

[S] *Fairly common side-effects are dizziness and confusion.*

A trade name is Parlodel.

brompheniramine
an ANTIHISTAMINE drug used to treat hay fever and perennial allergic rhinitis. A trade name is Dimotane Plus. **[0]**

Brompton cocktail
a mixture of alcohol, morphine and cocaine sometimes given to control severe pain in terminally ill people, especially those dying of cancer. The mixture was first tried at the Brompton Hospital, London and has given relief to thousands.

bromsulphthalein
a substance used in a liver function test. The rate of clearance of bromsulphthalein from the blood, after injection, is a measure of liver efficiency. The test is now largely replaced by enzyme tests.

Brufen
a trade name for IBUPROFEN. **[O]**

Brulidine
a trade name for a preparation containing
DIBROMOPROPAMIDINE. **[O]**

budesonide
a CORTICOSTEROID DRUG used in a nasal spray for
hay fever (allergic rhinitis) or as an inhalant for
asthma. It is also administered as a cream or
ointment for the treatment of eczema, psoriasis
and other kinds of dermatitis. Trade names are
Pulmicort (inhalant), Preferid (cream).

bufexamac
an NSAID administered externally in the form of a
cream for the treatment of skin inflammation and
to relieve itching. A trade name is Parfenac.

bumetanide
a quick-acting diuretic drug used to relieve the
fluid retention (oedema) occurring in heart failure,
kidney disease such as the nephrotic syndrome and

cirrhosis of the liver. or by injection. A trade name is Burinex.

bupivacaine
a long-acting local anaesthetic drug often used for nerve blocks, especially in epidural anaesthesia during childbirth and for the control of post-operative pain. A trade name is Marcaine.

buprenorphine
a powerful synthetic opiate pain-killing drug that binds to the body's opioid receptors. It acts for six to eight hours.

[»] *Buprenorphine is administered by mouth.*

[S] *Side-effects include drowsiness, nausea, dizziness and sweating.*

A trade name is Temgesic.

Burinex
a trade name for BUMETANIDE.

Buscopan
a trade name for HYOSCINE.

buselerin
a drug that simulated the action of the
gonadotrophin releasing hormone gonadorelin. A
trade name is Suprecur (women), Suprefact (men).

Buspar
a trade name for BUSPIRONE.

buspirone
a non-benzodiazepine anti-anxiety drug with slow
onset of effect.

busulphan
an anticancer drug used especially in the treatment
of chronic granulocytic leukaemia.

[S] *It is very toxic and can destroy the function of
the bone marrow unless its use is carefully
monitored. It can also cause widespread fibrosis of
the lungs.*

A trade name is Myleran.

Butacote
a trade name for PHENYLBUTAZONE.

Butazolidin
a trade name for PHENYLBUTAZONE.

Butazone
a trade name for PHENYLBUTAZONE.

butobarbitone
a barbiturate hypnotic drug of medium duration of action. A trade name is Soneryl.

butriptyline
a tricyclic drug used in the treatment of depression. A trade name is Evadyne.

butyrophenone drugs
a group of phenothiazine derivative drugs used in the treatment of schizophrenia. They act as dopamine receptor antagonists. The group includes HALOPERIDOL, triperidol and benperidol.

Cafergot
a trade name for a mixture of ERGOTAMINE and
CAFFEINE.

caffeine
one of the most popular and widely used drugs of
mild addiction. Caffeine is used, in the form of
coffee, tea and Cola-flavoured drinks, by about half
the population of the world. It elevates mood,
controls drowsiness, decreases fatigue and
increases capacity for work.

Caladryl
a trade name for a mixture of CALAMINE, camphor
and DIPHENHYDRAMINE. [O]

calamine
zinc carbonate, zinc silicate or zinc oxide. Calamine
is widely used as a bland, mildly astringent, skin
lotion. A little phenol (carbolic acid) is often added
for its itch-relieving properties. [O]

Calcicard
a trade name for diltiazem.

calciferol
vitamin D. A fat-soluble vitamin necessary for the absorption of calcium from the intestine. Deficiency causes rickets in infants and osteomalacia in adults.

Calcihep
a trade name for HEPARIN.

Calcimax
a trade name for CALCIUM.

calcipotriol
a vitamin D analogue drug administered as an ointment for the treatment of psoriasis. A trade name is Dovonex.

Calcitare
a trade name for calcitonin.

calcium channel blockers
drugs which interfere with the movement of dissolved calcium through cell membranes. Calcium is necessary for the contraction of muscles, and calcium ions must pass through special ion channels

in the membrane of cells if the muscles are to contract. Calcium channel blockers block this movement and so interfere with the action of the muscle fibres, relaxing the smooth muscle in the walls of arteries so that the blood pressure is reduced and the flow through the coronary arteries of the heart is improved.

They are valuable in angina pectoris and in reducing the oxygen consumption of the heart. Like many others, these drugs are broken down in the liver. About four hours after a dose, half the drug has gone.

Adalat (nifedipine) and Tildiem (diltiazem) are valuable in cases of spasm of the coronary arteries and can relieve angina. They are often used in conjunction with beta-blocker drugs.

Cordilox (verapamil), Clinium (lidoflazine) and Synadrine (prenylamine) are also helpful in cases of irregular heartbeat (cardiac arrhythmias).

[S] *These drugs do have side-effects including*

undue slowing of the heart, heart block, and low blood pressure.

calcium chloride

a calcium salt limited in its usefulness because of its irritating properties. It may be given by very slow intravenous injection and is sometimes used in cases of cardiac arrest.

calcium gluconate

a calcium salt commonly given by mouth as a calcium supplement in the treatment of rickets, osteomalacia and osteoporosis.

calcium lactate

a calcium salt used as a calcium supplement.

calcium oxalate

a calcium salt occurring in the urine, sometimes in such high concentration as to form urinary stones (calculi).

calcium sodium lactate

a combination of calcium and sodium lactates used

to supplement body calcium.

Calmazine
a trade name for TRIFLUOPERAZINE.

Calpol
a trade name for PARACETAMOL. **[O]**

Caltrate
a trade name for calcium.

Calvita
a trade name for a mixture of vitamins and
minerals.

Camcolit 250
a trade name for LITHIUM.

Camoquin
a trade name for AMODIAQUINE.

Canesten
a trade name for CLOTRIMAZOLE. **[O]**

cannabis
the hemp plant or its dried flowering leaves.

Cantil [W]
a trade name for mepenzolate.

Caplenal
a trade name for ALLOPURINOL.

Capoten
a trade name for CAPTOPRIL.

capreomycin
an ANTIBIOTIC drug derived from Streptomyces capreolus and used in the treatment of tuberculosis resistant to standard drugs such as RIFAMPICIN, ISONIAZID, ETHAMBUTOL and STREPTOMYCIN.

capsicum
cayenne pepper. Sometimes used as a counter-irritant to promote improved local blood flow in inflammation. Occasionally used in proprietary cough and indigestion mixtures.

captopril

an angiotensin converting enzyme inhibitor (ACE INHIBITOR) drug used in the treatment of heart failure and high blood pressure (hypertension).

Capurate

a trade name for ALLOPURINOL.

Carafate

a trade name for SUCRALFATE.

carbachol

a drug with acetyl choline-like properties of stimulating the parasympathetic nervous system. It is used to stimulate peristalsis in the intestine, to treat retention of urine and sometimes to treat glaucoma.

carbamazepine

a drug used in the control of epilepsy and especially to relieve or prevent the pain of trigeminal neuralgia. The trade name is Tegretol.

KEY

The symbol [O] indicates that the drug is either available over-the-counter or that an over-the-counter drug with the same active ingredient or ingredients is available.

The symbol [»] indicates the forms in which the drug can be taken.

The symbol [S] sets out side-effects.

The symbol [W] indicates a drug recently withdrawn. These drugs should not be used.

carbaryl
a drug administered in the form of a lotion or shampoo to kill head and pubic lice. A trade name is Carylderm, Clinicide.

carbenicillin
an ANTIBIOTIC of the penicillin group.

carbenoxolone
a drug used to promote healing in stomach and

duodenal ulcers. It has now been largely replaced
by drugs such as cimetidine and ranitidine.

carbidopa
a drug that prevents the breakdown of the drug
levodopa in the body and thus enhances its action
in Parkinson's disease. See also BENSERAZIDE.

carbimazole
an antithyroid drug that interferes with the
production of thyroid hormone and is used in the
treatment of hyperthyroidism.

carbimide, calcium
a drug that produces very unpleasant symptoms if
followed by alcohol. Like DISULFIRAM, it is
occasionally used to try to discourage drinking in
alcoholics.

Carbrital
a trade name for PENTOBARBITONE.

carbromal
a mild sedative and hypnotic drug.

[S] *It may cause skin rashes, especially if sensitive to bromine. The drug is now seldom used.*

Cardene
a trade name for NICARDIPINE.

Cardiacap
a trade name for PENTAERYTHRITOL TETRANITRATE.

Cardinol
a trade name for PROPRANOLOL.

Carylderm
a trade name for CARBARYL.

cascara sagrada
the 'sacred bark' of the cascara buckthorn tree Rhamnus purshiana, formerly used as a laxative.

castor oil
an oil derived from the poisonous seeds of the plant, Ricinus communis and formerly used to treat constipation.

Catapres
a trade name for clonidine, a drug used to treat high blood pressure. A stimulator of the alpha$_2$-adrenoceptor sites.

Cedocard
a trade name for ISOSORBIDE DINITRATE.

cefaclor
a broad-spectrum ANTIBIOTIC.

[»]*One of the CEPHALOSPORINS that can be taken by mouth.*

cefotaxime
a third-generation CEPHALOSPORIN ANTIBIOTIC active against Gram-negative organisms but not staphylococci.

cefuroxime
a second-generation CEPHALOSPORIN ANTIBIOTIC active against staphylococci and some Gram-negative organisms.

209

[»] *It must be given by injection.*

Celestone
a trade name for BETAMETHASONE.

centoxin
a bacterial endotoxin antibody administered by injection in cases of dangerous bacterial infection with overwhelming toxicity.

cephalexin
a CEPHALOSPORIN ANTIBIOTIC effective by mouth.

cephalosporins
a range of ANTIBIOTICS, chemically similar to penicillins. First obtained from a Cephalosporium fungus found in the sea near a sewage outflow, many semisynthetic forms have been developed. Their toxicity is low and they are effective against a wide range of organisms.

Ceporacin
a trade name for cephalocin, a CEPHALOSPORIN ANTIBIOTIC.

Ceporex
a trade name for cephalexin, a CEPHALOSPORIN
ANTIBIOTIC.

Cerubicin
a trade name for DAUNORUBICIN.

Cetavlon
a trade name for CETRIMIDE. **[0]**

cetrimide
a detergent antiseptic and cleaning substance used
in solution or as an ointment. A trade name is
Cetavlon. **[0]**

cetylpyridinium chloride
a local antiseptic and disinfectant used in some
proprietary cough medicines. **[0]**

chelating agent
any drug that combines with metal ions within the
body to form an insoluble chelate – a molecule
consisting of a ring of atoms of which one is a
metal. Chelating agents are thus valuable in

211

effectively removing from the body toxic metallic compounds or metallic salts present in excess.

Chemotrim
a trade name for CO-TRIMOXAZOLE.

Chendol
a trade name for CHENODEOXYCHOLIC ACID.

Chenocedon
a trade name for CHENODEOXYCHOLIC ACID.

chenodeoxycholic acid
a drug used in the treatment of cholesterol gallstones, which it gradually dissolves over a period of up to eighteen months.

[S] *A common side-effect is diarrhoea.*

Trade names are Chendol, Chenofalk, Chenocedon.

Chenodol
a trade name for CHENODEOXYCHOLIC ACID.

Chenofalk
a trade name for CHENODEOXYCHOLIC ACID.

Chinine
a trade name for QUININE.

Chloractil
a trade name for CHLORPROMAZINE.

chloral hydrate
a bitter substance used in solution as a sedative and hypnotic.

chlorambucil
a nitrogen-mustard drug used in the treatment of leukaemia and lymphomas including Hodgkin's disease.

chloramphenicol
an ANTIBIOTIC originally derived from the soil bacterium Streptomyces venezuelae.

[S] *It is highly effective in many serious conditions but has dangerous side-effects which limit its use.*

chlordiazepoxide
a benzodiazepine sedative and tranquillizer.

Millions are dependent on this drug and doctors are becoming increasingly concerned.

A trade name is Librium.

chlorhexidine
a disinfectant used in surgery for preoperative skin cleansing and for sterilizing instruments by soakage. A trade name is Hibitane. [O]

chlormethiazole
a sedative and anticonvulsant drug related to vitamin B_1 used in the management of the alcohol withdrawal syndrome.

Chlorocort
a trade name for eye drops containing CHLORAMPHENICOL and HYDROCORTISONE.

chloroethane
see ETHYL CHLORIDE.

chloroform
a heavy, colourless, volatile liquid once widely used as a pleasant and easy general anaesthetic.

It has been abandoned because of its tendency to cause cardiac arrest and other dangerous complications including delayed liver atrophy.

Chloromycetin
a trade name for CHLORAMPHENICOL.

chloroquine,
a drug used in the treatment of malaria, rheumatoid arthritis and lupus erythematosus.

chlorothiazide
a thiazide DIURETIC drug used to lower blood pressure. The thiazides have this effect mainly by relieving the blood of excess water but also by making the muscles in the vessel walls less responsive to noradrenaline.

chloroxylenol
antiseptic for local use. A trade name is Dettol. [O]

chlorpheniramine
an ANTIHISTAMINE drug used to treat hay fever, perennial allergic rhinitis and anaphylactic shock. A trade name is Piriton.

chlorpromazine,
a drug derived from phenothiazine used as an antipsychotic, a tranquillizer and to prevent vomiting (anti-emetic). The trade name is Largactil.

chlorpropamide
a drug used in the treatment of Type II (non-insulin dependency) diabetes.

[S] *It can cause severe and prolonged low blood sugar (hypoglycaemia) and facial flushing if alcohol is taken.*

chlortetracycline,
an ANTIBIOTIC obtained from the soil bacterium Streptomyces aureofaciens. The trade name is Aureomycin.

chlorthalidone

a DIURETIC drug of medium potency that increases the output of urine over a period of forty-eight hours.

Chlotride

a trade name for CHLOROTHIAZIDE.

cholagogue

a drug, such as dehydrocholic acid, that promotes the flow of bile.

cholecalciferol

vitamin D_3, the natural form of the vitamin, formed in the skin by the action of the ultraviolet component of sunlight on 7-dehydrocholesterol.

Choledyl

a trade name for CHOLINE THEOPHYLLINATE.

cholestyramine

a drug used in the treatment of hyperlipidaemia. It is an anion-exchange resin that binds bile acids so that they cannot be reabsorbed and are lost in the

217

stools. This stimulates the conversion of body cholesterol into more bile acids. A trade name is Questran.

choline

one of the B vitamins necessary for the metabolism of fats and the protection of the liver against fatty deposition. The important neuro-transmitter acetylcholine is formed from it.

choline theophyllinate

a drug used in the treatment of asthma. It is similar in its action to theophylline but less irritating and can be taken by mouth.

Cicatrin

a trade name for BACITRACIN and NEOMYCIN.

Cidomycin

a trade name for GENTAMICIN.

Cilamox

a trade name for AMOXICILLIN.

cimetidine

a histamine H_2 receptor antagonist drug used to limit acid production in the stomach in cases of peptic ulcer. The best known trade name is Tagamet.

cinchocaine

a powerful local anaesthetic drug.

cinchona

a south American tree, genus Cinchona, from the bark of which quinine is derived.

cinnarizine

a drug used to treat Ménière's syndrome.

clavulanic acid

a drug that interferes with beta-lactamase enzymes (penicillinases) that inactivate many penicillin-type ANTIBIOTICS, such as AMOXICILLIN. When taken in combination with the antibiotic, this drug can overcome drug resistance. Trade names of the combination: Augmentin, Timentin.

clemastine

an ANTIHISTAMINE drug used to treat hay fever and perennial allergic rhinitis. A trade name is Tavegil. [0]

clenbuterol

a beta-adrenergic agonist drug useful in the treatment of asthma. The drug is capable of causing a considerable increase in the bulk of voluntary muscle (hypertrophy) with an increase in force and a reduction in relaxation time. It is also valuable as means of preventing the atrophy of muscle, that has been deprived of its nerve supply, during the long period of nerve regeneration.

KEY

The symbol [O] indicates that the drug is either available over-the-counter or that an over-the-counter drug with the same active ingredient or ingredients is available.

The symbol [»] indicates the forms in which the drug can be taken.

The symbol [S] sets out side-effects.

The symbol [W] indicates a drug recently withdrawn. These drugs should not be used.

---

clindamycin
an ANTIBIOTIC drug that penetrates well into bone to treat osteomyelitis.

clinistix
a narrow strip of card impregnated with an enzyme that produces a purple colour when dipped into urine containing sugar. This is a convenient routine screening test for diabetes.

Clinitar
a trade name for a preparation containing COAL TAR. [O]

clinitest
a method of urine testing for sugar (glucose) using a tablet that is dropped into the urine in a test tube. This method gives a quantitative result by causing colour changes from green (0.5% glucose) to orange (2% glucose).

Clinoril
a trade name for SULINDAC.

clofazimine
a drug used to treat leprosy. It is effective in controlling the erythema nodosum reaction. A trade name is Lamprene.

clofibrate
a drug that lowers the blood cholesterol levels. A trade name is Atromid.

Clomid
a trade name for CLOMIPHENE.

clomiphene
a drug used to treat infertility by virtue of its ability
to stimulate the production of eggs from the
ovaries (ovulation). Multiple pregnancies often
result. A trade name is Clomid.

clomipramine
a tricyclic ANTIDEPRESSANT DRUG useful, also, in
phobic anxiety and obsessive states. A trade name
is Anafranil.

clonazepam
a BENZODIAZEPINE drug used to control epilepsy
and trigeminal neuralgia. A trade name is Rivotril.

clonidine
an alpha$_2$ adrenoreceptor stimulator (agonist) that
is effective in lowering blood pressure and
controlling some cases of migraine and
postmenopausal flushing. A trade name is Dixarit.

Stopping treatment may produce a dangerous rise in blood pressure.

clopamide
a thiazide diuretic drug. A trade name is Viskaldix.

clotrimazole
a drug effective against a wide range of fungi.

[»] *It is used in the form of creams, for local application.*

A trade name is Canesten. [0]

clove oil
an aromatic oil distilled from the flower buds of the clove tree, used mainly by dentists as a mild antiseptic and toothache reliever. Mixed with zinc oxide [0], it forms a widely used temporary dressing for a tooth cavity.

cloxacillin
a semisynthetic penicillin ANTIBIOTIC that resists the destructive penicillinase enzymes that some

staphylococci produce. The drug also resists degradation by stomach acid and so can be taken by mouth.

clozapine
a benzodiazepine antipsychotic drug used in the treatment of schizophrenia resistant to other drugs.

[S] *It is notable for the absence of tremors and repetitive movements (dyskinesias) in those taking it, but it may seriously affect white blood cell production by the bone marrow and may cause drowsiness, salivation, fatigue, dizziness, headache and urinary retention.*

A trade name is Clozaril.

coal tar
a complex mixture of organic substances, especially polycyclic hydrocarbons, derived from the distillation of coal. Although the action of this mixture is not well understood, coal tar preparations are used empirically to treat various

skin disorders such as eczema and psoriasis. [O]

cobalamin
vitamin B_{12}. The specific treatment for pernicious anaemia.

Cobutolin
a trade name for SALBUTAMOL.

cocaine
the main alkaloid of the bush Erythroxylon coca, introduced to medicine by Sigmund Freud. Cocaine was the first effective local anaesthetic drug, but is not now widely used in medicine, having been replaced by safer analogues. It is a major 'recreational' drug, producing a euphoria similar to that of AMPHETAMINE and has many undesirable behavioural and social effects.

Codalgin
a trade name for CODEINE and PARACETAMOL. [O]

Codate
a trade name for CODEINE.

codeine
an alkaloid derived from opium, used to control
moderate pain, to relieve unnecessary coughing
and to check diarrhoea. Codeine is not a drug of
addiction and is available without prescription.

Codelix
a trade name for CODEINE.

Codesol
a trade name for PREDNISOLONE.

Codiphen
a trade name for a mixture of ASPIRIN and
CODEINE. [O]

Codis
a trade name for a mixture of ASPIRIN and
CODEINE. [O]

codliver oil
an extract of the liver of the codfish, rich in
vitamins A and D.

Cogentin
a trade name for BENZTROPINE.

Colifoam
a trade name for HYDROCORTISONE. [0]

colistin,
an ANTIBIOTIC produced by the bacterium Bacillus colistinus and effective against Pseudomonas aeruginosa. It is used to sterilize the inside of the bowel and bladder and on the skin and external ear.

colocynth
a drastic purgative drug, no longer in use.

Cologel
a trade name for methylcellulose, used as a laxative.

Colomycin
a trade name for COLISTIN.

Combantrin
a trade name for PYRANTEL.

common cold remedies
drugs purporting to cure colds, but that actually do
no more than suppress symptoms. It is well known
in medical circles that if a cold is left untreated, it
lasts for about a week, but that if the most
effective known remedies are applied, it will last
for about seven days. Jokes of this kind are merely
a reflection of the fact that no practical remedy
exists which has any significant effect on most of
the two hundred or so strains of viruses that cause
the common cold.

Some, the rhinoviruses, can probably be controlled
by a large daily dose of alpha2-interferon, given as
a nasal spray, but this is very expensive and causes
nose bleeds.

Millions of pounds are spent every year on over-
the-counter common cold remedies, but in spite of
implied claims, none of these has anything but a
symptomatic effect. There are drugs which stop the

KEY

The symbol **[O]** indicates that the drug is either available over-the-counter or that an over-the-counter drug with the same active ingredient or ingredients is available.

The symbol **[»]** indicates the forms in which the drug can be taken.

The symbol **[S]** sets out side-effects.

The symbol **[W]** indicates a drug recently withdrawn. These drugs should not be used.

---

nose running and make it easier to breath, drugs which relieve the discomfort of the sore throat, even drugs which make you feel that a cold is not such a bad thing after all, but these are merely covering up the symptoms and the cold will still be there until the immune system gets the better of it.

Comox

a trade name for CO-TRIMOXAZOLE.

Compazine
a trade name for PROCHLORPERAZINE.

Concordin
a trade name for PROTRIPTYLINE.

Conova 30
an oral contraceptive containing ethinyloestradiol and ethynodiol.

Contac
a trade name for a mixture of ATROPINE, HYOSCINE, HYOSCYAMINE and PSEUDOEPHEDRINE.

co-proxamol
an ANALGESIC drug consisting of a combination of the drug paracetamol and the weakly narcotic drug dextropropoxyphene. Trade names: Distalgesic, Paxalgesic.

Corbeton
a trade name for OXPRENOLOL.

Cordarone X
a trade name for AMIODARONE.

Cordilox
a trade name for VERAPAMIL.

Corgard
a trade name for NADOLOL.

Corlan
a trade name for HYDROCORTISONE. **[0]**

Coro-Nitro
a trade name for nitroglycerine (GLYCERYL TRINITRATE).

Cortaid
a trade name for HYDROCORTISONE. **[0]**

Cortate
a trade name for CORTISONE.

Cortef
a trade name for HYDROCORTISONE. **[0]**

Cortelan
a trade name for CORTISONE.

corticosteroid drugs
drugs that simulate the action of the body's own
steroid hormones. The corticosteroids were first
isolated from the outer layer (cortex) of the
adrenal gland, where the hormone cortisol is
produced. A steroid is a member of the large
chemical group, related to fats, which includes
sterols such as cholesterol, bile acids, sex hormones,
many drugs and the adrenal cortex hormones.
Corticosteroid drugs are similar to the natural
corticosteroid hormones.

[»] *They have many uses and can be given by
injection, by mouth, as ointments or creams or as
eye or ear drops.*

They are powerful anti-inflammatory drugs,
prescribed for many conditions in which
inflammation may cause damage to the body.
These include inflammatory diseases of the bowel
such as regional ileitis (Crohn's disease) and

ulcerative colitis; joint inflammation such as rheumatoid arthritis; inflammation of arteries, as in temporal arteritis; inflammation in the eye (uveitis); asthma; hay fever (allergic rhinitis); and eczema.

They are used to suppress the immune responses which lead to the rejection of a donated organ transplant and are often life-saving in conditions of severe stress in which the production of natural hormones is inadequate. And they are given as hormone replacement therapy to people with disease of the adrenal glands (Addison's disease). Powerful drugs tend to have major side-effects and the corticosteroids, given in large dosage, are no exception. But a sense of proportion is necessary. Steroid skin ointments and creams, used occasionally, are unlikely to do any harm and, indeed, some of these are available without prescription.

[S] *Powerful steroids used on the skin can, however, cause atrophy and thinning.*

Steroids used in an inaler are also unlikely to have

anything other than local side-effects, as the dose is very small.

Steroids in high doses for long periods will inevitably cause some side-effects and these vary with the dose and the method of administration.

[S] Important side-effects include the suppression of the natural production of steroids so that stopping the treatment is dangerous; the reactivation of latent infection and an increased susceptibility to new infections; the breakdown of peptic ulcers; osteoporosis; diabetes; high blood pressure; excessive hairiness (hirsutism); glaucoma; and, rarely, cataract.

The decision to give long-term steroids to young children must be balanced against the fact that these drugs cause severe stunting of growth. It must be remembered that the same effect may be caused by serious childhood illnesses, for which steroids may be needed.

Because long-term treatment with cortico-steroids

suppresses the body's production of corticosteroid hormones by the adrenal glands, sudden withdrawal of the drugs is the equivalent of adrenal failure and may lead to collapse and death. For this reason all patients on long-term steroid treatment should carry a card indicating, in detail, the treatment they are having.

cortisol

a hormone produced by the adrenal cortex. Also called hydrocortisone.

cortisone

the first CORTICOSTEROID produced for treatment purposes. It is converted to hydrocortisone in the liver. It was used to treat rheumatoid arthritis, severe allergies, adrenal failure and other conditions but has been largely replaced by more powerful synthetic steroids.

Cortistab

a trade name for CORTISONE.

Corusic
a trade name for ALLOPURINOL.

Cosylan
a trade name for DEXTROMETHORPHAN. **[0]**

co-trimoxazole
an effective combination of the sulphonamide sulphamethoxazole and trimethoprim. The drug is useful in acute bronchitis, urinary infections, salmonella infections and in the treatment of typhoid carriers. Trade names are Septrin and Bactrim.

Coumadin
a trade name for WARFARIN.

cromoglycate, sodium
a drug used in allergies. It stabilizes the membrane of the mast cells that otherwise release histamine and other irritating substances when antibodies (IgE) and allergens (such as pollen grains) react on their surfaces.

Cuprofen
a trade name for IBUPROFEN. [O]

curarine
a poisonous alkaloid obtained from curare and used as a muscle relaxant or paralysant in general anaesthesia. It acts by competing with acetylcholine at the point at which motor nerves stimulate muscle fibres. The form used in anaesthesia is called tubocurarine.

cyanocobalamin
vitamin B_{12}. This vitamin is necessary for the normal metabolism of carbohydrates, fats and proteins, for blood cell formation and for nerve function. It is used in the treatment of pernicious anaemia and sprue.

Cyclidox
a trade name for DOXYCYCLINE

Cyclimorph
a trade name for morphine and cyclizine.

Cyclogyl
a trade name for eye drops containing
CYCLOPENTOLATE.

Cyclopane
a trade name for a mixture of PAPAVERINE,
ATROPINE and PARACETAMOL.

cyclopentolate
a drug used to dilate the pupils of the eyes for
purposes of examination of the retina and other
internal parts. A trade name is Mydrilate.

cyclophosphamide
a drug that substitutes an open chain hydrocarbon
radical for a hydrogen atom in a cyclic organic
compound (alkylating agent). It is used as an
anticancer drug for its alkylating action on the
guanine molecule in DNA. The margin between the
effective dose and the dangerous dose is narrow.
Side-effects include loss of hair, sterility, sickness
and vomiting and depression of blood formation
by the bone marrow. A trade name is Endoxana.

cyclopropane
a powerful, non-irritating anaesthetic gas. It has the disadvantages of causing heart irregularity in the presence of adrenaline.

cycloserine
a drug used to treat tuberculosis caused by organisms resistant to treatment by standard drugs such as RIFAMPICIN, ISONIAZID, ETHAMBUTOL and STREPTOMYCIN.

Cyclospasmol
a trade name for cyclandelate, a drug that helps to improve blood supply to any part of the body by relaxing the arteries.

cyclosporin
an important immunosuppressant drug that has greatly reduced the rate of rejection of grafted organs such as kidneys and hearts. It acts by interfering with the multiplication of immunocompetent T lymphocytes. A trade name is Sandimunn.

> **KEY**
>
> The symbol [O] indicates that the drug is either available over-the-counter or that an over-the-counter drug with the same active ingredient or ingredients is available.
>
> The symbol [»] indicates the forms in which the drug can be taken.
>
> The symbol [S] sets out side-effects.
>
> The symbol [W] indicates a drug recently withdrawn. These drugs should not be used.

Cyklokapron

a trade name for TRANEXAMIC ACID.

cyproheptadine

an ANTIHISTAMINE drug used to treat allergic disorders generally including itchy skin conditions.

[S] *Side-effects include stimulation of appetite, interactions with monoamine oxidase inhibitors and drowsiness.* A trade name is Periactin.

Cyprostat

a trade name for cyproterone.

Cytacon

a trade name for CYANCOBALAMIN.

Cytadren

a trade name for AMINOGLUTETHIMIDE.

Cytamen

a trade name for CYANCOBALAMIN.

cytarabine

an antimetabolite drug used in the treatment of acute leukaemia. It is a purine antagonist and acts by depriving cells of essential metabolic substances.

[S] *It causes sickness and vomiting, peptic ulcers and depression of bone marrow blood formation.*

cytotoxic drugs

anticancer drugs. Drugs which exert a more severely damaging or destructive effect on certain cells than on others. Usually the differentiation occurs on the basis of rapidity of reproduction and cytotoxic drugs are most active against cells, such as those in cancers, which are not restrained in their ability to multiply. They cannot avoid causing some damage to normal cells and consequently always have major side-effects.

Cytotoxic drugs are especially useful in the treatment of some forms of leukaemia, lymphomas and cancers of the testicle and ovary. They are often used as an additional safeguard after surgery or in conjunction with radiotherapy.

[S] *Unfortunately, they can cause damage to any rapidly growing group of cells, such as the lining of the bowel, the hair, the sex glands and the blood forming tissue in the bone marrow.*

[S] *Typical side-effects include nausea, vomiting, hair loss, sterility, anaemia and a tendency to bleeding. Treatment with these drugs is always accompanied by monitoring of the blood cell count.*

Cytotoxic drugs include chlorambucil, cyclophosphamide, lomustine, methotrexate, vinblastine, vincristine, adriamycin, bleomycin and nitrogen mustard.

Dactil
a trade name for piperidolate.

Daktarin
a trade name for MICONAZOLE.

Dalacin C
a trade name for CLINDAMYCIN.

Dalmane
a trade name for flurazepam.

danazole
a synthetic progestogen drug that inhibits secretion by the pituitary gland of the sex-gland stimulating hormone gonadotrophin. It is used to treat precocious puberty, breast enlargement in the male (gynaecomastia), excessively heavy menstrual periods (menorrhagia) and endometriosis. A trade

name is Danol.

Daneral-SA
a trade name for PHENIRAMINE.

Danocrine
a trade name for DANAZOLE.

Danol
a trade name for DANAZOLE.

Dantrium
a trade name for DANTROLENE.

dantrolene
a drug used to relieve muscle spasm in any spastic condition such as cerebral palsy, multiple sclerosis or spinal cord injury. It is taken by mouth or given by injection.

[S] *Liver damage sometimes occurs.*

A trade name is Dantrium.

Daonil

a trade name for GLIBENCLAMIDE.

dapsone

a drug to treat leprosy, but irregular use has led to the development of drug resistance. dapsone is also used in the treatment of dermatitis herpetiformis which may be associated with coeliac disease.

Daranide

a trade name for DICHLORPHENAMIDE.

Daraprim

a trade name for PYRIMETHAMINE.

daunorubicin

an ANTIBIOTIC drug that interferes with DNA synthesis and is used in the consolidation phase of the treatment of acute leukaemia.

DDAVP

see DESMOPRESSIN.

Deca-Durabolin
a trade name for nandrolone.

Decadron
a trade name for DEXAMETHASONE.

decongestant drugs
drugs used to shrink the congested and swollen
(oedematous) lining of the nose and so relieve
'stuffiness'. Decongestant drugs act on the alpha
adrenergic receptors in the nose lining, stimulating
them and so constricting the blood vessels
supplying the mucous membrane. The result is that
less fluid flows into the membrane and it becomes
less swollen.

[»]*These drugs may be applied as drops, inhalants
or sprays.*

Many decongestants have an adrenaline-like
action. Drugs which are used for this purpose
include ephedrine, amphetamine, phenylephrine,
tranazoline, oxymetazoline and xylometazoline.
Amphetamine was once a popular decongestant

but became too popular and was discontinued.

Many decongestants are highly effective in relieving nasal obstruction and reducing the thickness of the mucous membrane, but have the disadvantage that this effect is soon followed by 'rebound' recongestion. This limits their value and often leads to overuse so that adrenaline effects may be experienced – fast pulse, tremor, and physical and mental overactivity.

Friar's balsam is a long-established medication: a tincture of benzoin, made by dissolving crushed benzoin, aloes, tolu balsam and storax in alcohol. It is popular as an inhalant, but this ritual, although hallowed by tradition, is unsupported by evidence of any real therapeutic value.

See also Common cold remedies.

Decortisyl
a trade name for PREDNISOLONE.

Decrin
a trade name for a mixture of ASPIRIN and
CODEINE. [0]

Deltasolone
a trade name for PREDNISOLONE.

Demerol
a trade name for PETHIDINE (meperidine).

deodorizing drugs
drugs used to eliminate, mask or prevent
undesirable odours. Body deodorants are often
antiperspirant drugs combined with masking
perfumes and have little real deodorant action.
They work by simply reducing the amount of sweat
available for bacterial breakdown – the cause of
the body odour.

Real deodorants are highly porous substances, such
as the clay Fuller's earth, silica gel or activated
charcoal. These are all highly effective deodorants,
but are unsuitable for general use on the body.

```
KEY
The symbol [O] indicates that the drug is either
available over-the-counter or that an over-the-
counter drug with the same active ingredient or
ingredients is available.

The symbol [»] indicates the forms in which the
drug can be taken.

The symbol [S] sets out side-effects.

The symbol [W] indicates a drug recently
withdrawn. These drugs should not be used.
```

Antiseptics may deodorize by eliminating odour-
producing organisms. Hexachlorophene, a
powerful germicide, was, at one time, widely used
in deodorants. Unfortunately, it was found to cause
nervous system damage and is no longer used for
this purpose.

Depo-Medrone, Depo-Medrol
trade names for METHYLPREDNISOLONE used as a
depot injection.

Depo-Provera
a contraceptive, given by depot injection,
containing medroxyprogesterone.

Dequacaine
a trade name for BENZOCAINE and dequalinium in
lozenge form.

Dequadin
a trade name for dequalinium in lozenge form.

Deralin
a trade name for PROPRANOLOL.

Dermacort
a trade name for a HYDROCORTISONE skin
preparation. [0]

Dermazole
a trade name for ECONAZOLE.

Dermonistat
a trade name for MICONAZOLE.

Dermovate
a trade name for clobetasol, a powerful topical
steroid.

DES
see DIETHYLSTILBESTROL.

Deseril
a trade name for METHYSERGIDE.

desferrioxamine
an iron CHELATING AGENT used in iron overload
conditions or iron poisoning. A trade name is
Desferal.

designer drugs
modifications of existing psychoactive drugs so as
to produce seemingly new drugs not covered by
prohibitive legislation. Designer drugs are
produced in secret laboratories for profit and
without regard to their dangers.

desmopressin
a drug used in the treatment of diabetes insipidus.

Desmopressin, or DDAVP, is a long-acting analogue of the natural pituitary hormone vasopressin, which is deficient in this condition.

[»] *The drug is given in a nasal spray or in the form of nose drops.*

desogestrel
a progestogen drug used in various oral contraceptives, often in combination with an oestrogen drug.

dexamethasone
a synthetic CORTICOSTEROID drug used for its anti-inflammatory action and for its value in reducing oedema of the brain. A trade name is Decadron.

dexamphetamine
the dextrorotatory form of amphetamine sulphate, a drug sometimes used to treat narcolepsy, hyperactivity in children and as an ANALEPTIC in hypnotic poisoning. It is widely abused. A trade name is Dexedrine.

Dexedrine
a trade name for DEXAMPHETAMINE.

Dexmethasone
a trade name for DEXAMETHASONE.

dextromethorphan
an opioid drug, with little useful pain-killing action,
used to control persistent and unproductive cough.
[O]

dextropropoxyphene
a pain-killing drug similar to METHADONE. The
trade name is Doloxene and it is also dispensed in
combination with paracetamol, as Distalgesic.
Overdosage is one of the commonest causes of
death by poisoning, as absorption is rapid and
breathing is quickly paralysed. It is not much more
effective than CODEINE and some poisoning
experts think it should be withdrawn.

DF118
a trade name for dihydrocodeine tartrate.

Diabex
a trade name for METFORMIN.

Diabinese
a trade name for CHLORPROPAMIDE.

diacetylmorphine
heroin. See DIAMORPHINE.

Diaformin
a trade name for METFORMIN.

Diamicron
a trade name for GLICLAZIDE.

diamorphine
heroin. A semisynthetic morphine derivative 3,6-O-diacetylmorphine hydrochloride monohydrate. Its effects are the same as those of morphine, to which it is converted in the body, but it is much more soluble and is rapidly absorbed when taken by mouth. This is helpful when it is used in the control of severe terminal pain.

The manufacture of diamorphine, even for medical use, is illegal in almost all countries. It is still used medically in Britain.

Diamox
a trade name for acetazolamide, a drug used in the treatment of GLAUCOMA and sometimes in the treatment of epilepsy and periodic paralysis.

Diarrest
a trade name for a preparation of dicyclomine, an antispasmodic drug that relieves painful bowel cramps, and codeine phosphate.

Diatensec
a trade name for SPIRONOLACTONE.

Diazemuls
a trade name for DIAZEPAM.

diazepam
a long-acting BENZODIAZEPINE drug used to treat severe acute anxiety, delirium tremens, epilepsy and muscle spasms. It is also used as a pre-operative

medication (pre-medication). or injection. Trade
names: Diazemuls, Valium.

Dibenyline
a trade name for PHENOXYBENZAMINE.

dibromomannitol
a drug used in the treatment of chronic leukaemia.

dibromopropamidine
an antibacterial and fungistatic agent for external
use. **[0]**

dichloralphenazone
a hypnotic drug used for short periods for the
management of insomnia and sometimes to control
delirium. A trade name is Welldorm.

dichlorophen
an ANTHELMINTIC drug used to remove
tapeworms. A trade name is Antiphen.

dichlorphenamide
a DIURETIC drug with a short duration of action. It

257

is also used in the treatment of glaucoma. A trade name is Daranide.

diclofenac
a non-steroidal anti-inflammatory drug (NSAID) used in the treatment of rheumatoid arthritis and other painful conditions.

Diconal
a trade name for the powerful ANALGESIC DIPIPANONE.

dicoumarol
an oral anticoagulant drug now mainly used as a rat poison. Other more readily controllable coumarins, such as WARFARIN, are now used.

Dicynene
a trade name for ETHAMSYLATE.

didanosine
a drug that interferes with the action of the enzyme reverse transcriptase by means of which the human immunodeficiency virus (HIV), the cause

of AIDS, is able to convert its RNA into DNA that can incorporate itself into the human DNA and replicate in the host cell. The drug is used in the attempt to prolong the live of sufferers from AIDS. There is no evidence that the drug can cure AIDS.

didronel

a drug used to improve mineralization of bone in women suffering from osteoporosis after the menopause, especially those who have already suffered fractures. A trade name is Didronel PMO (post-menopausal osteoporosis).

dienoestrol

a synthetic oestrogen drug. A trade name is Hormofemin.

diethylcarbamazine

a drug used to treat the parasitic worm diseases filariasis and onchocerciasis. The drug kills both the microfilaria and the adult worms but may provoke severe reactions when the worms die. A trade name is Banocide.

diethylpropion
an AMPHETAMINE-like drug used to reduce appetite to try to help in the management of obesity. Trade names are Apisate and Tenuate Dospan.

diethylstilbestrol
A synthetic female sex hormone. This is now restricted in use to the treatment of certain cancers of the prostate and the breast.

If given to pregnant women it can cause cancer in the female offspring. In Britain, about 7500 pregnant women were given the drug and five unequivocal cases of clear cell cancer occurred in their daughters. There were six other possible cases. In the USA 361 cases of clear cell cancer have occurred to date in women whose mothers had been given the drug.

diflunisal
a non-steroidal pain-killing and anti-inflammatory drug (NSAID). It is a derivative of salicylic acid and is used to control symptoms in osteoarthritis and

---

KEY

The symbol [O] indicates that the drug is either available over-the-counter or that an over-the-counter drug with the same active ingredient or ingredients is available.

The symbol [»] indicates the forms in which the drug can be taken.

The symbol [S] sets out side-effects.

The symbol [W] indicates a drug recently withdrawn. These drugs should not be used.

---

other painful conditions. A trade name is Dolobid.

digitalis
a drug used in the treatment of heart failure. It increases the force of contraction and produces a slower, more regular pulse. The drug is derived from the purple foxglove Digitalis purpurea and is usually given in the form of DIGOXIN.

digoxin
a valuable heart drug derived from the white foxglove Digitalis lanata. It is the most widely used of the DIGITALIS heart drugs and is a member of the group of cardiac glycosides.

dihydrofolate reductase inhibitors
drugs that interfere with the conversion of folic acid to its active form in the body, such as pyrimethamine, trimethoprim, triamterene and methotrexate. When such drugs are necessary, folate deficiency is treated with folinic acid rather than folic acid. Methotrexate potentiates the effects of other dihydrofolate reductase inhibitors.

Dilantin
a trade name for the ANTICONVULSANT phenytoin.

Dimatab
a trade name for a mixture of PARACETAMOL and PSEUDOEPHEDRINE. [0]

Dimelor
a trade name for ACETOHEXAMIDE.

dimenhydrinate
an ANTIHISTAMINE drug used mainly to control
motion sickness. The trade name is Dramamine.

dimercaprol
British AntiLewisite (BAL). A drug that takes up
toxic metal ions from the body and can be life-
saving in poisoning with lead, arsenic, gold,
mercury, antimony, bismuth and thallium. It was
developed during the First World War in the course
of a search for antidotes to poison war gases,
particularly the arsenical Lewisite.

dimethicone
a silicone preparation used externally to retain skin
moisture in cases of undue drying and to protect it
against irritating external agencies. It is commonly
used to prevent nappy rash in babies. Trade names:
Siopel, Conotrane. [O]

dimethindine maleate
an ANTIHISTAMINE drug used to treat hay fever,
urticaria and other allergic conditions. Trade names
are Fenostil Retard, Vibrocil.

Dimotane
a trade name for BROMPHENIRAMINE. **[0]**

Dindevan
a trade name for PHENINDIONE.

dinoprost
a prostaglandin F2a drug used to terminate
pregnancy or to expel a fetus that has died.

[»] *Taken by mouth or as a vaginal tablet or gel.*

A trade name is Prostin F2 alpha.

Dioctyl
a trade name for the lazative docusate.

diphenhydramine
an ANTIHISTAMINE drug now used mainly for its
sedative properties in children and for travel
sickness. A trade name is Benadryl. **[0]**

diphenoxylate
a drug related to PETHIDINE and with a codeine-

like action on the bowel. It is used to treat diarrhoea. It is sold, mixed with a little ATROPINE, under the trade name of Lomotil.

diphosphonates

a group of drugs that interfere with crystal formation and are used to relieve the symptoms of Paget's disease of bone.

diprophylline

a drug similar to AMINOPHYLLINE used to relax bronchial muscle spasm in asthma and to improve the action of the heart. A trade name is Noradran.

Diprosone

a trade name for BETAMETHASONE in a preparation for external use.

dipyridamole

a drug used to reduce platelet stickiness and thus the risk of stroke in people having transient ischaemic attacks. Aspirin is more effective, but sometimes cannot be safely taken. A trade name is Persantin.

Disalcid
a trade name for salsalate, a drug of similar composition and properties to aspirin.

Disipal
a trade name for ORPHENADRINE.

disodium cromoglycate
see CROMOGLYCATE.

disopyramide
a drug used to prevent or control disturbances of heart rhythm. A trade name is Dirythmin.

Disprin
a trade name for ASPIRIN. [O]

Distaclor
a trade name for cephaclor, a CEPHALOSPORIN ANTIBIOTIC.

Distalgesic
a trade name for a mixture of PARACETAMOL and DEXTROPROPOXYPHENE.

Distamine
a trade name for PENICILLAMINE.

distigmine
an anticholinesterase drug used to treat
myasthenia gravis. A trade name is Ubretid.

disulfiram
a drug that interferes with the normal metabolism
of alcohol so that a toxic substance, acetaldehyde,
accumulates. This causes flushing, sweating,
nausea, vomiting, faintness, headache, chest pain
and sometimes convulsions and collapse. The trade
name is Antabuse.
*It is sometimes used to discourage drinking, but is
not without danger.*

dithranol
a drug used in the treatment of psoriasis. It is an
ANTIMITOTIC agent and acts to discourage
overgrowth of epidermal cells. A trade name is
Exolan.

Dithrolan

a trade name for DITHRANOL and SALICYLIC ACID.

ditiocarb

the sodium salt of diethyldithiocarbamate, a powerful ANTI-OXIDANT and CHELATING AGENT that has been used to treat immune deficiency conditions, such as AIDS. It appears to be effective in reducing the incidence of opportunistic infections and cancers in HIV positive people.

Diuresal

a trade name for FRUSEMIDE.

diuretic drugs

drug that causes an increased output of urine. Various heart, kidney and liver disorders can cause water to accumulate abnormally in the tissue spaces of the body, or within some of the body cavities. Fluid in the tissues is called oedema and fluid in the cavities is called an effusion. Tissue fluid accumulation tends to affect the dependent parts of the body –the ankles and lower back and the lower parts of the lungs.

Oedema can interfere with body function –
especially in the lungs – and causes unwanted
weight gain and other disadvantages. Oedema is
always an indication of some other disorder and, if
possible, the cause should be corrected. Often, this
will clear up the oedema, but it is often necessary
to get rid of the excess fluid in a more direct
manner. This is the job of the diuretic drugs.

Normally, the kidneys filter very large volumes of
water out of the blood. If all this water entered the
urine, we would quickly die of dehydration, so
most of it is reabsorbed back into the blood.
Diuretics act on certain parts of the kidneys to
prevent some of this reabsorption of water and
allow a proportion of it to pass out in the urine.
When they do this, the blood becomes
concentrated and the excess fluid in the tissues is
drawn into it, thus relieving the oedema.

Diuretics are very effective. Lasix (Frusemide) or
Burinex bumetanide) acts within an hour and the
effect on the kidneys lasts for about six hours.
Large quantities of urine may be produced – up to

10 litres in a day.

Too rapid loss of fluid may reduce the blood volume undesirably and can be dangerous. There may also be danger from the undue loss of potassium from the body, but doctors are aware of this danger and, if necessary, give potassium tablets to make up losses.

[»] Diuretics are nearly always taken by mouth, but sometimes, in an emergency, they may be given by injection. In long-term conditions causing oedema they are given in a dosage just sufficient to keep the fluid from accumulating in the tissues.

In addition to those mentioned, diuretic drugs include Aldactone (spironolactone), Aprinox (bendrofluazide), Diamox (acetazolamide), Edecrine (ethacrynic acid), Hydrosaluric (hydrochlorothiazide), Moduretic (amiloride) and Navidrex (cyclopenthiazide). They act in slightly different ways on the kidneys, but they all have the same useful effect.

Diurexan
a trade name for xipamide, a thiazide diuretic
drug.

Dixarit
a trade name for CLONIDINE.

dobutamine
a drug used to assist in the management of heart
failure. It increases the force of the contraction
(inotropic agent) of the muscle of the ventricles
and improves the heart output.
[»] *It may be given by continuous intravenous drip.*

Dolmatil
a trade name for sulpiride, a drug used to treat
psychotic disorders.

Doloxene
a trade name for DEXTROPROPOXYPHENE.

domiphen bromide
an antiseptic used in throat lozenges. A trade name
is Bradosol Plus. [0]

KEY

The symbol [O] indicates that the drug is either available over-the-counter or that an over-the-counter drug with the same active ingredient or ingredients is available.

The symbol [»] indicates the forms in which the drug can be taken.

The symbol [S] sets out side-effects.

The symbol [W] indicates a drug recently withdrawn. These drugs should not be used.

---

domperidone

a drug used to control nausea and vomiting. An anti-emetic. It acts to close the muscle ring at the upper opening of the stomach (the cardia) and to relax the ring at the lower opening (the pylorus). or suppository. Trade names: Evoxin, Motilium.

Donnalix

a trade name for a mixture of ATROPINE, HYOSCINE and HYOSCYAMINE.

dopamine
a natural body catecholamine neuro-transmitter derived from dopa that acts on receptors throughout the body, especially in the limbic system and extrapyramidal system of the brain and in the arteries and the heart. The effects vary with the concentration. It is used as a drug to improve blood flow to the kidneys and to increase the strength of contraction of the heart in heart failure, shock, severe trauma and septicaemia. See also dopamine receptor agonists, dopamine receptor antagonists.

dopamine receptor agonists
drugs that have an effect on the body similar to that of dopamine. They include bromocriptine and lisuride and are used to treat Parkinson's disease, acromegaly, overproduction of the hormone prolactin, and to suppress or prevent milk secretion.

dopamine receptor antagonists
drugs that compete with dopamine to occupy and block the dopamine receptor sites in the body. They

include the phenothiazines, butyrophenones and
thioxanthenes used to treat psychosis.

Dopram
a trade name for DOXAPRAM.

Dormonoct
a trade name for loprazolam, a BENZODIAZEPINE
hypnotic drug.

doxapram
a drug that stimulates breathing and consciousness.
An ANALEPTIC drug similar in its action to
NIKETHAMIDE. A trade name is Dopram.

doxazosin
a selective alpha-adrenergic blocker drug used to
treat high blood pressure. A trade name is Cardura.

doxorubicin
an ANTIBIOTIC, also known as Adriamycin, that
interferes with the synthesis of DNA and is thus
useful as an anticancer agent.

[S] *It has many side-effects including loss of hair, sickness and vomiting, interference with blood production and heart damage.*

doxycycline
a tetracycline ANTIBIOTIC drug, deoxytetracycline, that is well absorbed when taken by mouth, even after food.

Doxylin
a trade name for DOXYCYCLINE.

Dozic
a trade name for HALOPERIDOL.

Dramamine
a trade name for DIMENHYDRINATE. A drug used to control motion sickness. It may cause sleepiness.

Drapolene
an antiseptic skin cream containing CETRIMIDE and benzalkonium chloride. **[0]**

Droleptan

a trade name for DROPERIDOL.

Dromoran

a trade name for the ANALGESIC levorphanol.

droperidol

a butyrophenone antipsychotic drug that causes emotional quietening and a state of mental detachment. It is sometimes used as a premedication before surgery. A trade name is Droleptan.

Dryptal

a trade name for FRUSEMIDE.

Ducene

a trade name for DIAZEPAM.

Duogastrone

a trade name for CARBENOXOLONE.

Duphalac

a trade name for LACTULOSE.

Durabolin [W]
a trade name for NANDROLONE, an ANABOLIC
STEROID.

Duractin
a trade name for CIMETIDINE.

Duromine
a trade name for PHENTERMINE.

Duromorph
a trade name for morphine.

Duvadilan
a trade name for isoxsuprine, a drug that widens
blood vessels and relaxes the muscles of the womb.

Dyazide
a trade name for TRIAMTERENE.

Dymadon
a trade name for PARACETAMOL. **[0]**

Dynese
a trade name for magaldrate, an antacid
combination of aluminium hydroxide and
magnesium hydroxate. [0]

Dyspamet
a trade name for CIMETIDINE.

Dytac
a trade name for triamterene, a DIURETIC drug that
does not lead to loss of potassium from the body.

Ebufac
a trade name for IBUPROFEN.

econazole
a broad-spectrum antifungal drug used to treat
ringworm and candidiasis. Trade names: Ecostatin,
Pevaryl.

ecothiopate
a powerful cholinergic drug of the
organophosphate anticholinesterase group, used in
the form of eye drops to cause prolonged

constriction of the pupil. The drug is useful in the treatment of some cases of glaucoma and strabismus. A trade name is Phospholine iodide.

Ecotrin
a trade name for ASPIRIN. [O]

ecstasy
a popular name for the drug 3,4-methylenedioxymet-amphetamine (MDMA), a hallucinogenic amphetamine with effects that are a combination of those of LSD and amphetamine.

This drug can precipitate a persistent paranoid psychosis.

Edecril, Edecrin
a trade name for ETHACRYNIC ACID.

edetate
ethylene-diamine-tetra-acetic acid (EDTA). Dicobalt EDTA is an antidote to cyanide, administered intravenously as soon as possible after poisoning.

edrophonium
a drug used to test for myasthenia gravis. A good response usually confirms the diagnosis.

EDTA
ethylene-diamine-tetra-acetic acid, a CHELATING AGENT.

Efcortelan
a skin ointment containing HYDROCORTISONE. **[O]**

eflornithine
a new drug recently approved by the World Health Organization for the treatment of African sleeping sickness (trypanosomiasis). and by intravenous injection. A trade name is DMFO.

Efudix
a trade name for a preparation of FLUOROURACIL for external application.

Elantan
a trade name for ISOSORBIDE MONONITRATE.

KEY
The symbol [O] indicates that the drug is either available over-the-counter or that an over-the-counter drug with the same active ingredient or ingredients is available.

The symbol [»] indicates the forms in which the drug can be taken.

The symbol [S] sets out side-effects.

The symbol [W] indicates a drug recently withdrawn. These drugs should not be used.

Elavil
a trade name for AMITRIPTYLINE.

Elyzol
a trade name for METRONIDAZOLE.

emetine
an alkaloid derived from ipecacuanha sometimes used in the treatment of amoebiasis. It has now been largely replaced by the safer

METRONIDAZOLE.

enalapril
an ANGIOTENSIN CONVERTING ENZYME (ACE) INHIBITOR drug with useful action over twenty-four hours. The trade name is Innovace.

Endep
a trade name for AMITRIPTYLINE.

Enduron [W]
a trade name for the DIURETIC methylclothiazide.

enflurane
a volatile drug which is used to induce and maintain general anaesthesia.

enoxacin
a quinolone ANTIBIOTIC drug.

enolic acids
the group of non-steroidal anti-inflammatory drugs (NSAIDs) that includes the pyrazolones phenylbutazone and azapropazone and the oxicam

piroxicam.

enoximone
an inotropic drug used in heart failure to increase the force and output of the heart. A trade name is Perfan.

Epanutin
a trade name for the ANTICONVULSANT phenytoin.

ephedrine
a drug with a similar action to adrenaline but with a more stimulant effect on the nervous system, causing tremor, anxiety, insomnia and undue alertness. It is used to treat allergic conditions and asthma. Ephedrine nasal drops decongest a swollen nose lining. [O]

Epilim
a trade name for SODIUM VALPROATE.

epinephrine
adrenaline. Epinephrine is the favoured medical usage in the USA, but the term adrenaline is in

popular use. ad and renal are Latin for 'on' and 'kidney'. The corresponding terms in Greek are epi and nephron.

epoprostenol

prostacyclin. A powerful inhibitor of clumping of blood platelets and thus of blood clotting. It is used with heart-lung (cardiopulmonary bypass) machines and artificial kidneys (dialysis machines) to preserve the platelets in the blood being pumped through them. Epoprostenol also widens (dilates) arteries.

Equagesic

a trade name for a mixture of the anti-anxiety drug meprobamate, aspirin and ethoheptazine.

Equanil

a trade name for the anti-anxiety drug meprobamate.

ergocalciferol

vitamin D_2. This is produced in the body by the action of ultraviolet light on ergosterol. Vitamin D is necessary for the normal mineralization of bone.

Deficiency leads to rickets in growing children and bone softening (osteomalacia) in adults.

ergometrine
an ergot derivative drug used to promote contractions of the muscle of the womb (uterus). This can be valuable, after the baby is born, to close off the site of separation of the after-birth (placenta) and prevent postpartum haemorrhage. It is sometimes given when delivery of the baby is almost accomplished. A trade name is Syntometrine.

ergotamine
a drug that causes widened (dilated) arteries to narrow. It is thus useful in the treatment of migraine.

[S] *Overdosage is dangerous.*

A trade name is Femergin.

Ergotrate
a trade name for ERGOMETRINE.

Erymax
a trade name for the broad-spectrum ANTIBIOTIC erythromycin.

eserine
an anticholinesterase drug sometimes used to constrict the pupil and treat glaucoma.

Esidrex [W]
a trade name for HYDROCHLOROTHIAZIDE.

Esidrex-K
a trade name for HYDROCHLOROTHIAZIDE with potassium.

ethacrynic acid
a loop DIURETIC drug. A drug that acts on the tubules in the kidneys to interfere with the reabsorption of water and thus greatly increase the output of urine. A trade name is Edecrin.

ethambutol
a drug used, ideally in combination with other drugs, in the treatment of tuberculosis.

Ethambutol can cause damage to the optic nerves and if persisted with after vision is affected can cause blindness.

A trade name is Myambutol.

ethamsylate
a drug that reduces bleeding from small blood vessels and is used to treat excessive menstruation (menorrhagia). A trade name is Dicynene.

ethanol
the chemical name for ethyl alcohol, the main constituent of alcoholic drinks.

ethinyloestradiol
a powerful synthetic oestrogen drug that can be taken by mouth and is widely used as a component of oral contraceptives. Trade names are Anovlar, Controvlar, Gynovlar, Microgynon and Minovlar.

ethionamide
a drug used in the treatment of leprosy or in cases of tuberculosis resistant to other drugs.

ethisterone
a progestogen drug used to treat premenstrual
tension (PMT) and menstrual disorders. As
norethisterone, it is also a component of oral
contraceptives. A trade name is Micronor.

ethosuximide
an anti-epileptic drug used in the management of
absence attacks (Petit mal).

*It has no effect against major epilepsy and may
cause nausea and drowsiness.*

A trade name is Zarontin.

etoposide
an anticancer drug derived from a plant poison
epipodophyllotoxin. It is used chiefly in the
maintenance treatment of acute leukaemia after
remission has been achieved and the bone marrow
has recovered.

Eudemine
trade name for the hypoglycaemic drug diazoxide.

Euglucon
a trade name for GLIBENCLAMIDE.

Eugynon
an oral contraceptive containing
ETHINYLOESTRADIOL and LEVONORGESTREL.

Euhypnos
a trade name for TEMAZEPAM.

Eumovate
a trade name for the CORTICOSTEROID
clobetasone.

Eurax
a trade name for crotamiton used to treat scabies.

evening primrose oil
a drug used in the treatment of allergic skin disease
(atopic eczema).

Exolan [W]
a trade name for DITHRANOL.

KEY

The symbol [O] indicates that the drug is either available over-the-counter or that an over-the-counter drug with the same active ingredient or ingredients is available.

The symbol [»] indicates the forms in which the drug can be taken.

The symbol [S] sets out side-effects.

The symbol [W] indicates a drug recently withdrawn. These drugs should not be used.

---

factor VIII
a protein (globulin) necessary for the proper clotting of the blood. The absence of Factor VIII causes haemophilia but it can be isolated from donated blood and given to haemophiliacs to control their bleeding tendency.

Fansidar
a trade name for a mixture of PYRIMETHAMINE and SULFADOXINE.

Fargo
a trade name for an aerosol spray of LIGNOCAINE.

Farlutal
a trade name for MEDROXYPROGESTERONE.

Fasigyn
a trade name for TINIDAZOLE.

Fedrine
a trade name for EPHEDRINE.

Fefol
a trade name for a mixture of FOLIC ACID and IRON.

Feldene
a trade name for PIROXICAM.

Femodene
an oral contraceptive containing ETHINYLOESTRADIOL and GESTODENE.

Fenamine
a trade name for PHENIRAMINE.

Fenbid
a trade name for IBUPROFEN. **[0]**

fenbufen
a non-steroidal anti-inflammatory drug (NSAID)
used to relieve inflammation and the resulting pain
and stiffness. A trade name is Lederfen.

fenclofenac
a non-steroidal anti-inflammatory drug (NSAID).
See ANALGESIC DRUGS.

fenfluramine
a drug used in the management of obesity. It is
thought to work by producing a sense of having
eaten enough (satiety) rather than by suppressing
appetite.

fenoprofen
a non-steroidal anti-inflammatory drug (NSAID).
See ANALGESIC DRUGS.

fenoterol

a beta2-agonist, adrenaline-like drug that is valuable in the management of asthma while having comparatively little effect on the heart. Its action is similar to that of SALBUTAMOL. A trade name is Berotec.

Fenox

a trade name for nasal drops containing PHENYLEPHRINE.

fentanyl

a powerful, short-acting narcotic pain killer (ANALGESIC). A trade name is Sublimaze.

Fentazin

a trade name for PERPHENAZINE.

Feospan

a trade name for an IRON preparation.

Fergon

a trade name for an IRON preparation.

Ferritard
a trade name for an IRON preparation.

Ferrocap F
a trade name for FOLIC ACID and IRON.

ferrous gluconate
an iron compound used in the treatment of iron-deficiency anaemia.

ferrous sulphate
a bitter, greenish crystalline compound of iron used in the treatment of iron-deficiency anaemia.

Ferrum H
a trade name for an IRON preparation.

Fersamal
a trade name for an IRON preparation used to treat anaemia.

fibrinase
Factor XIII, an enzyme in the blood that catalyzes the formation of side links between fibrin

molecules so as to create a mesh of polymerized fibrin that stabilizes the blood clot. Fibrinase is also known as the fibrin-stabilizing factor. See also Factor VIII, IX, XII.

fibrinolytic drugs

a group of drugs capable of breaking down the protein fibrin which is the main constituent of blood clots. They are thus able to disperse dangerous blood clots (thromboses) that have formed within the circulation. They include streptokinase, alteplase, anistreplase and urokinase.

finasteride

a drug used to reduce the size of the prostate gland so as to help men suffering urinary difficulty from enlargement of the gland. Finasteride interferes with the action of a chemical activator (enzyme) that converts the sex hormone testosterone to dihydrotestosterone. It is the latter that causes the prostate to enlarge. The drug causes a significant decrease in obstruction symptoms and an increased urinary flow.

[S] *Side-effects include some reduction of sex drive and decreased volume of ejaculate.*

A trade name is Proscar.

FK 506

a new drug that interferes with the action of the immune system and can be used to prevent rejection of grafted organs. FK506 has also been used to treat allergic skin conditions and psoriasis.

[S] *Side-effects include damage to the kidneys.*

Flagyl

a trade name for METRONIDAZOLE.

flecainide

a drug used to control irregularity of the heartbeat.

[»] *It is taken by mouth.*

[S] *Possible side-effects include nausea, vomiting, dizziness, vertigo, jaundice, visual disturbances and nerve damage.*

A trade name is Tambocor.

Flopen
a trade name for FLUCLOXACILLIN.

flosequinan
a new drug that acts on the smooth muscle of
arteries and veins to cause both to relax and widen.
This greatly reduces the load on the heart in
patients with heart failure without affecting the
blood supply to the various parts of the body.

[S] *Side-effects include headache, dizziness and
palpitations. The drug is still being evaluated.*

Floxapen
a trade name for FLUCLOXACILLIN.

Fluanxol
a trade name for FLUPENTHIXOL.

flucloxacillin
a semisynthetic penicillin ANTIBIOTIC, readily
absorbed when taken by mouth and effective

against organisms that produce penicillin-
destroying enzymes (beta-lactamases). A trade
name is Floxapen. Magnapen.

fluconazole
an antimycotic drug used to treat candidiasis
(thrush) in any part of the body, externally or
internally. A trade name is Diflucan.

flucytosine
a drug used to treat fungus infections within the
body. It can be taken by mouth and is effective
against cryptococcosis, chromoblastomycosis and
candidiasis.

fludrocortisone
a steroid drug with a minor anti-inflammatory
action but with a powerful sodium-retaining effect,
similar to that of aldosterone. It is thus useful in
the treatment of Addison's Disease, to replace
aldosterone. A trade name is Florinef.

flumazenil
a benzodiazepine antagonist drug, used in

anaesthesia to reverse the effects of benzodiazepine drugs on the nervous system. A trade name is Anexate.

flunitrazepam
a benzodiazepine drug used for the short-term treatment of insomnia. A trade name is Rohypnol.

Fluorigard
a trade name for fluoride.

Fluoroplex
a trade name for FLUOROURACIL.

fluorouracil
a pyrimidine anticancer drug.

fluoxetine
an ANTIDEPRESSANT drug that acts by prolonging the action of the neuro-transmitter 5-hydroxytryptamine (5HT or serotonin). It is is a selective serotonin re-uptake inhibitor which is taken by mouth. This drug is currently being taken by some 10 million people, mainly in the USA, and

is said to be the most popular psychoactive drug in the history of pharmacology. It has attracted a great deal of attention as a 'mood brightener' and enhancer of optimism. It is claimed to be capable of altering personality for the better.

[S] *Possible side-effects include nausea, diarrhoea, insomnia, anxiety, violent outbursts, fever, skin rash and convulsions.*

A trade name is Prozac.

flupenthixol
a thioxanthene antipsychotic drug used to treat schizophrenia and other psychoses.

[»] *It is taken by mouth or given by injection.*

[S] *Possible side-effects include sedation and involuntary movements.*

Trade names are Depixol and Fluanxol.

KEY

The symbol [O] indicates that the drug is either available over-the-counter or that an over-the-counter drug with the same active ingredient or ingredients is available.

The symbol [»] indicates the forms in which the drug can be taken.

The symbol [S] sets out side-effects.

The symbol [W] indicates a drug recently withdrawn. These drugs should not be used.

---

fluphenazine

a phenothiazine derivative drug used in the treatment of psychotic conditions.

[»]*It can be given by injection for long-term effect.*

The Trade name is Modecate.

Flurets

a trade name for a fluoride preparation.

301

fluvoxamine
an ANTIDEPRESSANT DRUG that acts by prolonging the action of the neuro-transmitter 5-hydroxytryptamine (5HT).

folic acid
a vitamin of the B group originally derived from spinach leaves, necessary for the synthesis of DNA and red blood cells. Deficiency causes megaloblastic anaemia. The drug is used successfully to prevent neural tube defects, such as spina bifida, in babies. Folic acid is plentiful in leafy vegetables and liver but is also produced by bacteria in the bowel and absorbed into the circulation. Deficiency may occur after ANTIBIOTIC treatment.

Folicid, Folicin [W]
trade names for FOLIC ACID.

Fortagesic
a trade name for a mixture of PARACETAMOL and PENTAZOCINE.

Fortral
a trade name for PENTAZOCINE.

foscarnet
an antiviral drug active against herpes viruses,
including cytomegaloviruses, that resist acyclovir,
especially in patients with AIDS. A trade name is
Foscavir.

framycetin
an ANTIBIOTIC drug used externally for skin
infections or as eye or ear drops. Trade names are
Sofradex and Soframycin.

Framycort
a trade name for a mixture of HYDROCORTISONE
and FRAMYCETIN.

Framygen
a trade name for FRAMYCETIN.

frusemide
a drug that causes an increased output of urine (a
diuretic) so as to relieve the body of unwanted

retained water (oedema). Frusemide acts on the kidney tubules where it interferes with chloride and sodium reabsorption from the dilute filtered urine. This prevents reabsorption of water into the blood and the result is a large volume of dilute urine. Trade names are Lasix, Frusetic and Frusid.

Frusetic
a trade name for FRUSEMIDE.

Frusid
a trade name for FRUSEMIDE.

Fucidin
a trade name for FUSIDIC ACID.

Fulcin
a trade name for GRISEOFULVIN.

Furacin
a trade name for NITROFURAZONE.

Furadantin
a trade name for nitrofurantoin, an antibacterial

used in the treatment of the urinary tract.

fusidic acid
a steroid ANTIBIOTIC used in the form of sodium
fusidate against penicillin-resistant (beta-
lactamase-producing) staphylococci. It has no value
against streptococci and is usually given in
conjunction with another ANTIBIOTIC such as
FLUCLOXACILLIN.

Fybogel
a trade name for ISPHAGULA.

gamma globulin
a protein, one of the five classes of
immunoglobulins (antibodies). Gamma globulin, or
immunoglobulin G (IgG), is the most prevalent and
provides the body's main antibody defence against
infection. For this reason it is produced
commercially from human plasma and used for
passive protection against many infections,
especially hepatitis, measles and poliomyelitis.

ganciclovir
an antiviral drug similar in composition to the DNA base guanine used to treat severe cytomegalovirus infections, mainly in patients with AIDS. A trade name is Cymevene.

Garamycin
a trade name for GENTAMICIN.

Gastreze
a trade name for a mixture of ALUMINIUM HYDROXIDE, MAGNESIUM TRISILICATE and the foam-dispersing agent simethicone. [0]

Gastrobrom
a trade name for a mixture of MAGNESIUM TRISILICATE, MAGNESIUM HYDROXIDE, MAGNESIUM CARBONATE and chalk (calcium carbonate).

Gastromax
a trade name for METOCLOPRAMIDE.

Gelusil
a trade name for a mixture of ALUMINIUM HYDROXIDE, MAGNESIUM HYDROXIDE and the foam-dispersing agent simethicone. **[0]**

gemeprost
a prostaglandin drug, administered as a vaginal pessary to terminate pregnancy. It causes powerful contractions of the womb at any stage of pregnancy. A trade name is Cervagem.

Genisol
a trade name for a shampoo containing COAL TAR. **[0]**

gentamicin
an aminoglycoside ANTIBIOTIC used mainly for the treatment of serious gram negative infections. Otherwise, Gentamicin is used topically for external infections, such as those of the eye or ear.

[S] *In large dosage it can cause tinnitus, deafness and kidney damage.*

Genticin
a trade name for GENTAMICIN.

Geriplex
a trade name for a multivitamin preparation.

gestodene
an oestrogen/progestogen oral contraceptive. A trade name is Femodene, Minulet.

glibenclamide
a sulphonylurea drug, similar in action and effect to CHLORPROPAMIDE, and used in the treatment of maturity onset (Type II) diabetes.

gliclazide
a sulphonylurea oral hypoglycaemic drug used in the treatment of Type II diabetes. A trade name is Diamicron.

Glimel
a trade name for GLIBENCLAMIDE.

glipizide
a sulphonylurea oral antidiabetic drug used in maturity-onset (Type II) diabetes. It operates by stimulating secretion of insulin by the pancreas and is administered by mouth. A trade name is Glibenese, Minodiab.

glucocorticoids
CORTISOL and other similar hormones produced by the outer zone (cortex) of the adrenal gland. The glucocorticoids suppress inflammation and convert amino acids from protein breakdown into glucose, thus raising the blood sugar levels. Their effect is thus antagonistic to that of INSULIN.

Glucophage
a trade name for METFORMIN.

Glucotard
a trade name for GUAR GUM.

glutaraldehyde
a substance used in solution to treat warts on the sole of the foot (plantar warts).

KEY

The symbol [O] indicates that the drug is either available over-the-counter or that an over-the-counter drug with the same active ingredient or ingredients is available.

The symbol [»] indicates the forms in which the drug can be taken.

The symbol [S] sets out side-effects.

The symbol [W] indicates a drug recently withdrawn. These drugs should not be used.

Glutarol

a trade name for GLUTARALDEHYDE.

glyceryl trinitrate

a drug highly effective in controlling the pain of angina pectoris. It is best taken in a tablet that is allowed to dissolve under the tongue and the pain is usually relieved in two to three minutes. Nitrates have a powerful action in widening (dilating) arteries, including the coronary arteries, thus improving the blood supply to the heart muscle.

Glyconon
a trade name for TOLBUTAMIDE.

Glymese
a trade name for CHLORPROPAMIDE.

glymidine
a sulphonylurea drug used in the treatment of non-insulin dependent diabetes. Like the other sulphonylureas, such as TOLBUTAMIDE and CHLORPROPAMIDE it is taken by mouth and reduces the blood sugar (oral hypoglycaemic drug).

gold salts
drugs such as auranofin or sodium aurothiomalate, used to treat rheumatoid arthritis. These are effective in slowing progress of the disease, especially in early cases.

[S] *Side-effects, such as mouth and tongue inflammation, itching, liver and kidney damage and blood disorders, are common.*

gold treatment
the use of gold salts, such as sodium
aurothiomalate, to treat rheumatoid arthritis.
These are effective in slowing progress of the
disease, especially in early cases.

[S] *Side-effects, such as mouth and tongue
inflammation, itching, liver and kidney damage
and blood disorders, are common.*

gonadorelin
the gonadotrophin-releasing hormone that
prompts the production of the hormone that
causes the sex glands to secrete their hormones.

gramicidin
an ANTIBIOTIC used externally in ointments and
creams, often in conjunction with NEOMYCIN and
FRAMYCETIN. It is too toxic for internal use.

Graneodin
a trade name for an ointment containing
GRAMICIDIN and NEOMYCIN.

griseofulvin
an antifungal drug derived from a Penicillium
mould that concentrates in the outer layers of the
skin and in the nails and is thus useful in the
treatment of 'ringworm' (tinea) infections. Skin
infections settle quickly, but tinea of the nails
requires treatment for months.

Griseostatin
a trade name for GRISEOFULVIN.

Grisovin
a trade name for GRISEOFULVIN.

guaiphenesin
a product of beechwood tar used as an expectorant
in many proprietary cough remedies.

guanethidine sulphate
a drug used in the treatment of high blood
pressure (hypertension). Trade names are Ismelin
and Ganda.

guar gum

an edible natural material with the property of binding carbohydrates in the intestine and reducing the rate of absorption so as to prevent a sudden increase in blood sugar. This is helpful in diabetes.

Guarem

a trade name for GUAR GUM.

Guarine

a trade name for GUAR GUM.

Gyne-Lotremin

a trade name for a vaginal preparation containing CLOTRIMAZOLE. [0]

Gyno-Daktarin

a trade name for MICONAZOLE.

Gyno-Pevaryl

a trade name for ECONAZOLE.

Gynovlar 21

an oral contraceptive containing
ETHINYLOESTRADIOL and NORETHISTERONE.

H_2 receptor antagonists

drugs that block the action of histamine on
receptors, mainly in the stomach, concerned with
the secretion of acid. Histamine is a powerful and
important hormone found in most body tissues in
inactivated form, mainly in the mast cells, and
released as a result of cell injury, either physical or
allergic (immunological). It has various actions,
causing smooth muscle, including that in the walls
of the air tubes of the lungs (bronchi) to contract,
arteries to dilate, capillaries to leak, skin to itch and
the lining of the stomach to secrete acid. There are
two kinds of histamine receptors – H_1 and H_2. H_1
receptor antagonists block the effects of histamine
produced as a result of allergic or other reactions
and are called ANTIHISTAMINE DRUGS. The H_2
receptor antagonists operate mainly in the stomach
lining and to a lesser extent in the walls of the
arteries.

H_2 receptor antagonists have revolutionized the treatment of stomach and duodenal ulcers by virtue of their action in blocking the secretion of acid. This important class of drugs includes Tagamet (cimetidine) and Zantac (ranitidine).

They are so effective that great care must be taken to ensure a correct diagnosis before using them as they can actually, for a time, relieve the symptoms of cancer of the stomach. They do not, of course, have any effect on the growth of cancer, and what may seem like successful treatment may lead to dangerous delay.

These drugs are also valuable in the management of heartburn (reflux oesophagitis), stress ulcers in people with severe burns and the Zollinger-Ellison syndrome.

[S] *There are few side-effects apart from the possible concealment of stomach cancer. These are minor and include diarrhoea or constipation, tiredness, headache, muscle pain, and slowing of the heart.*

316

[S] *Cimetidine has a weak antagonistic effect on the male sex hormones and may cause enlargement of the breasts in men and even impotence. Ranitidine does not have this effect.*

Halcion
a trade name for TRIAZOLAM.

Haldol
a trade name for HALOPERIDOL.

Haliborange
a trade name for a preparation containing vitamins A, D and C.

hallucinogenic drugs
drugs that cause hallucination. Most are derived from plants such as the desert peyote cactus, Lophophora williamsii from which mescaline is derived, the psilocybin-containing 'sacred mushrooms' and the seeds of the morning glory flower, which contains lysergic acid.

[S] *These drugs can precipitate a psychosis in*

predisposed people.

haloperidol
a butyrophenone drug used in the treatment of
psychiatric disorders. It is similar in its effects to the
PHENOTHIAZINE derivative drugs. A trade name is
Serenace.

halothane
a pungent, volatile, non-inflammable liquid
anaesthetic agent. Halothane is a powerful drug
that induces anaesthesia in a concentration of less
than 1 per cent.

[S] *Severe liver damage occurs very occasionally,
usually after a second exposure to the drug in a
sensitized subject.*

A trade name is Fluothane.

Hamarin
a trade name for ALLOPURINOL.

Harmogen
a trade name for PIPERAZINE.

Headclear
a trade name for a mixture of PARACETAMOL,
PSEUDOEPHEDRINE and CHLORPHENIRAMINE. [O]

heparin
a complex polysaccharide organic acid found
mainly in lung and liver tissue. Heparin is thought
to bind to thrombin and antithrombin in plasma
thereby assisting in their combination and
interfering with the cascade of reactions that end
in blood clotting (coagulation). Heparin is widely
used as an anticoagulant. From the Greek hepar,
the liver.

heroin
see DIAMORPHINE.

Herpid
a trade name for IDOXURIDINE.

hexachlorophane
a bactericidal agent used in soaps for skin cleansing.
A chlorinated phenol. A trade name is Phisohex.

Hexopal
a trade name for NICOTINIC ACID.

Hibitane
a trade name for CHLORHEXIDINE.

Histryl
a trade name for diphenylpyraline.

HMG CoA reductase inhibitors
drugs that interfere with the synthesis of
cholesterol by the liver and are used to reduce
abnormally high blood cholesterol levels. They
include lovastatin, simvastatin and pravastatin.

Hormonin
a trade name for the hormone oestradiol.

Humulin
a trade name for human INSULIN.

KEY

The symbol [O] indicates that the drug is either available over-the-counter or that an over-the-counter drug with the same active ingredient or ingredients is available.

The symbol [»] indicates the forms in which the drug can be taken.

The symbol [S] sets out side-effects.

The symbol [W] indicates a drug recently withdrawn. These drugs should not be used.

Hydopa
a trade name for the ANTIHYPERTENSIVE drug methyldopa.

hydralazine
a drug that causes arteries to widen (vasodilatation) and can be used as an adjunct to the treatment of high blood pressure (hypertension) by more conventional means. It is seldom used alone. A trade name is Apresoline.

hydrochlorothiazide
a drug used to increase the output of urine so as to relieve the body of surplus water. A thiazide DIURETIC drug. A trade name is Esidrex.

hydrocortisone
a natural steroid hormone derived from the outer layer (cortex) of the adrenal gland. The drug CORTISONE is converted into hydrocortisone in the liver. Hydrocortisone has anti-inflammatory and sodium-retaining properties. A trade name is Hydrocortone.[0]

Hydrocortisyl
a trade name for HYDROCORTISONE.[0]

Hydromet
a trade name for a mixture of HYDROCHLOROTHIAZIDE and the ANTIHYPERTENSIVE drug methyldopa.

Hydrosaluric
a trade name for HYDROCHLOROTHIAZIDE.

hydrotalcite
an antacid drug used to treat mild dyspepsia. It is found in several proprietary indigestion remedies. **[0]**

hydroxocobalamin
vitamin B$_{12}$. This is the specific treatment for pernicious anaemia and is highly effective unless neurological damage has already occurred. A trade name is Cobalin-H.

hydroxyzine
an ANTIHISTAMINE drug used to treat itching, nettle rash and as a sedative and to control vomiting. A trade name is Atarax.

Hygroton
a trade name for the DIURETIC drug chlorthalidone.

hyoscine
Scopolamine. A drug structurally related to ATROPINE and having similar properties. Trade names are Omnopon and Buscopan.

hyoscyamine
an ATROPINE-like drug used to relax smooth muscle spasm, as in colic, and for its sedative effect.

hypnotic drugs
drugs used to induce sleep in people with insomnia. They are also called sedatives or soporifics, and act to depress the action of the whole nervous system, especially that of the surface (cortex) of the brain – the seat of consciousness. Hypnotics include chloral hydrate, bromide salts, barbiturates, none of which are now commonly used, and the benzodiazepine drugs, which are used in great quantity. Chloral hydrate is still sometimes used to sedate sleepless children, but ANTIHISTAMINES, which also have a sedative effect, are more commonly given for this purpose.

[S] *Hypnotics in large dosage cause coma, interfere with normal breathing, reduce the blood pressure and body temperature and abolish reflex activity. Habituation, the acquisition of tolerance, and addiction with withdrawal symptoms are all common results of long-term use and this is now generally deprecated by doctors. Hypnotic drugs are potentially dangerous to life and are often used in suicide attempts. The automatic prescription of hypnotic drugs in response to a complaint of insomnia is bad medicine and it is necessary to take time to analyze the cause of the insomnia and deal with it directly. If hypnotics are used at all, they should be used sparingly and only for short periods. Millions are addicted to hypnotic drugs.*

Hypovase
a trade name for PRAZOSIN.

hypromellose
a preparation of METHYL CELLULOSE used in eye drops.

Hypurin
a trade name for INSULIN.

ibuprofen
a pain-killing (ANALGESIC) drug with anti-inflammatory properties, useful in mild rheumatic

and muscular disorders and in the relief of
menstrual pain. A trade name is Brufen.

idoxuridine
a drug effective against Herpes simplex viruses.
Idoxuridine is chemically very similar to thymidine,
a substance used nutritionally by the virus, which it
replaces. It has now been largely dispaced by
Acyclovir (Zovirax)

ifosfamide
an alkylating agent used as an anticancer drug.

Ilotycin
a trade name for the ANTIBIOTIC erythromycin.

Imferon
a trade name for an IRON preparation.

imidazole drugs
a class of antifungal and antibacterial drugs
effective against a wide range of bacteria and
fungi. The group includes metronidazole (Flagyl),
mebendazole, thiabendazole, clotrimazole

(Canesten), ketoconazole and miconazole. They administered by mouth or externally as creams.

imipramine
a widely used tricyclic ANTIDEPRESSANT DRUG. A trade name is Tofranil.

Imodium
a trade name for LOPERAMIDE.

Imunovir
a trade name for INOSINE PRANOBEX.

Imuran
a trade name for AZATHIOPRINE.

Inderal
a trade name for PROPRANOLOL.

Indocid
a trade name for INDOMETHACIN.

Indolar
a trade name for INDOMETHACIN.

indomethacin
a non-steroidal pain-killing (ANALGESIC) and anti-inflammatory drug (NSAID) of the indole acetic acid group. Trade names are Indocid, Artracin and Indolar.

indoramin
an alpha-adrenergic blocker drug used to treat high blood pressure. A trade name is Baratol, Doralese.

Indur
a trade name for ISOSORBIDE MONONITRATE.

Infacol
a trade name for DIMETHICONE. [0]

Inflam
a trade name for IBUPROFEN. [0]

Initard
a trade name for a slow acting INSULIN.

Inosine Pranobex
isoprinosine. A drug that enhances the efficiency of the immune system by increasing the number of T cells and enhancing the activity of natural killer cells. Trials in HIV-positive people suggest this drug could delay AIDS.

Insulatard
a trade name for a slow acting INSULIN.

insulin
a peptide hormone produced in the beta cells of the Islets of Langerhans in the pancreas. Insulin facilitates and accelerates the movement of glucose and amino acids across cell membranes. It also controls the activity of certain enzymes within the cells concerned with carbohydrate, fat and protein metabolism. Insulin production is regulated by constant monitoring of the blood glucose levels by the beta cells. Deficiency of insulin causes diabetes. Insulin preparations may be in the 'soluble' form for immediate action or in a 'retard' form for prolonged action.

Intal
a trade name for SODIUM CHROMOGLYCATE

Intraval
a trade name for sodium thiopentone.

Intron A
a trade name for interferon.

Intropin
a trade name for DOPAMINE.

iodine
a halogen element which, in small quantities, is an essential component of the diet. Iodine is poisonous in excess and is sometimes used in an alcoholic or aqueous potassium iodide solution as an antiseptic. The radioactive isotope, iodine 131, is extensively used for thyroid imaging and thyroid function tests.

iodoform
a yellowish iodine compound, containing about 96 per cent iodine, used as an antiseptic.

Ipral
a trade name for TRIMETHOPRIM.

iproniazid
an ANTIDEPRESSANT DRUG. A trade name is
Marsilid.

iron
an element essential for the formation of
haemoglobin. Lack of iron leads to iron-deficiency
anaemia. Iron is provided in a variety of chemical
forms for the treatment of anaemia.

[»] *Iron is usually taken by mouth. In urgent cases,
or if oral therapy fails, iron can be given by
injection.*

Isogel
a trade name for isphagula.

isometheptene
a sympathomimetic drug used in the treatment of
migraine. A trade name is Midrid.

isoniazid
a drug used in the treatment of tuberculosis.

[S] *The drug occasionally produces side-effects such as skin rash and fever, and rarely nerve involvement.*

A trade name is Rifater.

isophane insulin
a form of insulin modified by adsorption on to a protein molecule protamine so as to act for up to about twelve hours with delayed onset of action. Trade names are Neuphane, Insulatard and Humulin I.

isoprenaline
an air-tube widening (bronchodilator) and heart-stimulating drug used in the treatment of asthma and heart block. It is commonly taken by inhalation from an inhaler. Trade names are Aleudrin and Medihaler-iso.

Isoptin
a trade name for VERAPAMIL.

Isopto Tears
a trade name for artificial tears containing
HYPROMELLOSE.

Isopto Carpine
a trade name for PILOCARPINE eye drops in
HYPROMELLOSE.

isosorbide mono-, di- and trinitrate
drugs used to prevent angina pectoris and in the
treatment of heart failure. Trade names are Elantan
and Cedocard.

Isotard
a trade name for INSULIN.

isotretinoin
a drug related to vitamin A and used in the
treatment of severe acne that has failed to respond
to other measures. A trade name is Roaccutane.

isphagula husk
a bulking agent used to treat constipation,
diverticulitis and irritable bowel syndrome. Trade
names: Colven, Fybogel.

ivermectin
a drug used to kill microfilaria in the treatment of
onchocerciasis.

Jectofer
an iron preparation given by intramuscular
injection for the treatment of anaemia.

Kabikinase
a trade name for STREPTOKINASE.

kanamycin
a broad spectrum aminoglycoside ANTIBIOTIC
derived from a oil actinomycete. Kanamycin is
active against gram negative organisms but is now
largely replaced by Gentamicin. The
aminoglycosides can cause deafness, tinnitus and
kidney damage.

kaolin
a fine clay powder used as a suspension mixture in
the treatment of diarrhoea and sometimes as a
kind of mud poultice to apply local heat.

Kaopectate
a trade name for KAOLIN.

Keflex
a trade name for CEPHALEXIN.

Kemadrin
a trade name for PROCYCLIDINE.

Kemicetine
a trade name for the ANTIBIOTIC chloromycetin.

Kenalog
a trade name for TRIAMCINOLONE.

ketamine
a drug used by anaesthetists to produce
insensitivity to pain, mental and physical. A trade
name is Ketalar.

ketoconazole
an imidazole antifungal drug.

ketoprofen
a drug in the non-steroidal anti-inflammatory
(NSAID) and pain-killing (ANALGESIC) group. A
trade name is Orudis.

ketotifen
a drug that prevents the release of histamine and
other irritating substances from mast cells in
allergic conditions. Its action is similar to that of
CROMOGLYCATE but has the disadvantage of
causing drowsiness. A trade name is Zaditen.

Kiditard [W]
a trade name for QUINIDINE.

Konakion
a trade name for vitamin K (phytomenadione).

labetalol
a combined alpha- and beta-blocking drug,
sometimes found to be more effective in the

treatment of high blood pressure (hypertension)
than beta-blockers. Trade names are Labrocol and
Trandate.

Labrocol
a trade name for LABETALOL.

lachesine
a drug sometimes used to widen (dilate) the pupils
in people sensitive to ATROPINE.

lactofelicine
an ANTIBIOTIC derived from the protein lactofeline
in human milk. It is a single peptide and has been
found to be selectively effective against various
bacteria that cause diarrhoea and food poisoning,
especially Listeria species and Escherichia coli.

lactulose
a disaccharide sugar that acts as a gentle but
effective LAXATIVE DRUG. It is not absorbed or
broken down but remains intact until it reaches the
colon where it is split by bacteria and helps to
retain water, thereby softening the stools. Trade

names are Duphalac and Lactulose.

laetrile

a substance, amygdalin, derived from the seeds of
bitter almonds, apricots and other fruit, that has
been claimed to be effective in treating cancer. It is
said to yield a cyanide-containing compound,
mandelonitrile, under the action of enzymes said to
be more plentiful in cancers than in normal tissue.
There is no medically acceptable evidence that
laetrile has any value in the treatment of cancer.

lamotrigine

a new anticonvulsant drug used in the control of
epilepsy. A trade name is Lamictal.

Lanoxin

a trade name for DIGOXIN.

Laractone

a trade name for SPIRONOLACTONE.

Laraflex

a trade name for NAPROXEN.

Largactil
a trade name for CHLORPROMAZINE.

Larodopa
a trade name for the ANTIPARKINSONISM drug
levodopa.

Lasix
a trade name for FRUSEMIDE.

Lasma
a trade name for THEOPHYLLINE.

latamoxef
a CEPHALOSPORIN ANTIBIOTIC active against many
Gram-negative bacilli. A trade name is Moxalactam.

Latycin
a trade name for a TETRACYCLINE eye ointment.

laudanum
a solution of crude opium in alcohol (tincture of
opium). The alkaloids of opium are now refined
and separated and prescribed as specific drugs.

Laudanum was once casually recommended for a wide range of conditions.

laxative drugs
drugs used to treat constipation. Laxatives are popular, extensively taken and usually unnecessary. In spite of modern enlightenment, there is still a general belief that a calamity awaits anyone who fails to empty his or her bowels at least once a day. This belief is without foundation. Some people have a bowel motion three times a day, others three times a week. Some even less often. All are normal. Constipation can cause symptoms but they are neither harmful nor, as is often the result of the absorption of 'toxins' from the bowel. The 'toxin' theory is pure imagination.

Trouble with the bowels is more often caused by laxatives than cured. Many people, thinking that a daily bowel action is essential to health, severely abuse their lower intestines with laxatives, suppositories and enemas. This response to an imaginary disorder can produce a real one.

The best laxative is dietary fibre and plenty of this will ensure adequate bulk in the stools. The diet should be adjusted so as to replace refined carbohydrate with foods containing much vegetable fibre – fruit, vegetables and bran-containing cereals, such as 'All-Bran'. Bran is left when flour is extracted from cereals. It contains much cellulose vegetable fibre which can take up large quantities of water and it should always be accompanied by a good fluid intake. It is hard to eat too much bran. Such a diet will produce bulky, soft stools and regular motions. People prefer to buy expensively packaged bulking agents containing methyl cellulose, which has much the same effect, apart from the price. Isogel is made from psyllium seeds and contains mucilage which, like bran cellulose and methyl cellulose, also swells and bulks up with water.

For very occasional use other, more active laxatives, are reasonably safe. These include wetting agents such as dioctyl and poloxamer 188, lubricants such as liquid paraffin, and osmotic agents like Epsom, Glauber or Rochelle salts, which are not absorbed but remain in the bowel, retaining and attracting water and thereby increasing the bulk of the stools. Lactulose, which functions in the same way, is popular. With all of these, plenty of water should be drunk.

Irritant laxatives, like castor oil, senna, cascara and so on are best avoided and should not be used on a regular basis.

Enemas may be needed for the ill and the debilitated, but should be used under medical supervision.

Ledercort

a trade name for TRIAMCINOLONE.

Lederfen

a trade name for FENBUFEN.

Lentard

a trade name for INSULIN.

Lente insulin
a trade name for INSULIN.

Lethidrone
a trade name for NALORPHINE.

Leukeran
a trade name for CHLORAMBUCIL.

levallorphan
a morphine-related drug that acts as a morphine antagonist and is used to treat morphine poisoning, especially when this is causing dangerous depression of respiration. A trade name is Lorphan.

levamisole
an drug used to remove roundworms. It has also been found to have an effect in stimulating the immune system by increasing T-cell responsiveness and encouraging the activity of phagocyte cells (polymorphonuclear leucocytes and macrophages). It is effective in rheumatoid arthritis.

levonorgestrel
a synthetic female sex hormone similar in effect to
progesterone and used mainly as an oral
contraceptive. Irregular vaginal bleeding, breast
tenderness, nausea and headache. Trade names:
Microval, Neogest.

Levophed
a trade name for NORADRENALINE.

Libanil
a trade name for GLIBENCLAMIDE.

Librax, Libraxin
trade names for a mixture of CHLORDIAZEPOXIDE
and the atropine-like, sympathetic nervous system
blocking drug clidinium bromide.

Librium
a trade name for CHLORDIAZEPOXIDE.

Lidocaine
LIGNOCAINE or Xylocaine.

Lidothesin
LIGNOCAINE or Xylocaine.

lignocaine
a widely used local anaesthetic drug which is also
used by intravenous injection in the treatment or
prevention of acute disorders of heart rhythm such
as ventricular tachycardia and ventricular
fibrillation.

Limbritol [W]
a trade name for a mixture of AMITRIPTYLINE and
CHLORDIAZEPOXIDE.

Lincocin
a trade name for LINCOMYCIN.

lincomycin
an ANTIBIOTIC acting mainly on gram positive
organisms. A trade name is Lincocin.

lindane
an insecticide drug used externally to kill parasites
such as lice and the scabies mite Sarcoptes scabei. A

trade name is Esoderm, Lorexane.

Lingraine
a trade name for ERGOTAMINE.

Lioresal
a trade name for BACLOFEN.

lipid-lowering drugs
drugs used to reduce the levels of fats in the blood.
Constant high levels of fats (lipids), such as
cholesterol, in the blood are associated with a
tendency to the serious arterial disease of
atherosclerosis. Lipid-lowering drugs are no
substitute for a healthy, low-fat diet, but are
especially valuable in cases of genetically-induced
high lipid levels (familial hyperlipidaemia). These
drugs work in different ways. Most of the body
cholesterol is synthesized in the liver, and some
drugs interfere with the enzymes which do this.
Others interfere with the absorption of cholesterol-
containing bile salts from the intestine. Low levels
of bile salts in the blood prompts the liver to
convert more cholesterol into bile.

[S] *The side-effects of lipid-lowering drugs include diarrhoea, nausea and an increased tendency to form gallstones.*

Liquifilm Tears
a trade name for artificial tears containing polyvinyl alcohol.

Liskonum
a trade name for LITHIUM.

Litarex
a trade name for LITHIUM.

Lithicarb
a trade name for LITHIUM.

lithium
an element, the lightest known solid, used as the citrate or carbonate for the control of manic depressive states. Lithium is also used as the succinate in ointments for the treatment of seborrhoeic dermatitis and in shampoos for the control of dandruff.

lobeline
a mixture of alkaloids with action similar to nicotine. Lobeline is derived from plants of the Lobelia genus and has been used as a respiratory stimulant, but is of little medical importance.

Locoid
a trade name for HYDROCORTISONE. [O]

Loestrin
an oral contraceptive containing ETHINYLOESTRADIOL and NORETHISTERONE.

lofepramine
a drug used in the treatment of depression. or injection. A trade name is Gamanil.

Logynon
an oral contraceptive containing ETHINYLOESTRADIOL and LEVONORGESTREL.

Lomotil
a combination of diphenoxylate and atropine used to treat diarrhoea.

loop diuretics

drugs, including FRUSEMIDE and bumetanide, that cause a large output of water in the urine by affecting reabsorption of sodium and chloride in the loop of Henle tubules in the kidneys.

loperamide

a synthetic narcotic analogue drug used to control mild diarrhoea. A trade name is Imodium.

loprazolam

a long-acting benzodiazepine drug administered by mouth. A trade name is Loprazolam.

Lopressor

a trade name for the beta-blocker metoprolol.

loratadine

an ANTIHISTAMINE drug used to treat hay fever and perennial allergic rhinitis.

[S] *Possible side-effects include headache, fatigue and nausea.*

KEY

The symbol **[O]** indicates that the drug is either available over-the-counter or that an over-the-counter drug with the same active ingredient or ingredients is available.

The symbol **[»]** indicates the forms in which the drug can be taken.

The symbol **[S]** sets out side-effects.

The symbol **[W]** indicates a drug recently withdrawn. These drugs should not be used.

A trade name is Clarityn.

lorazepam
a benzodiazepine tranquillizer drug similar to Valium (DIAZEPAM). A trade name is Ativan.

Lotremin
a trade name for CLOTRIMAZOLE. **[O]**

lovastatin
see HMG CoA REDUCTASE INHIBITORS.

Ludiomil
a trade name for the ANTIDEPRESSANT
maprotiline.

Lugacin
a trade name for GENTAMICIN.

Madopar
a proprietary drug containing a mixture of a
dopamine precursor and an inhibitor of the
enzyme, dopa decarboxylase, that breaks down
dopamine. Madopar is used to treat the form of
Parkinsonism that sometimes follows encephalitis
(post-encephalitic Parkinsonism).

Magnapen
a mixture of the penicillin ANTIBIOTICS, AMPICILLIN
and FLUCLOXACILLIN.

magnesium carbonate
a mild antacid drug used to treat dyspepsia. A

351

trade name is Actonorm.

magnesium hydroxide
an antacid and laxative drug. A trade name is Milk
of Magnesia.

magnesium sulphate
a drug used by mouth or by enema to treat
constipation; by local application in a paste or
poultice to draw water from wounds; and by
injection to treat magnesium deficiency. A trade
name is Kest.

magnesium trisilicate
a drug used as an antacid in the treatment of
dyspepsia. A trade name is Actonorm.

Magnoplasm
a trade name for MAGNESIUM SULPHATE.

Maloprim
a mixture of PYRIMETHAMINE and DAPSONE used
in the treatment of malaria to eliminate the liver
cycle (exo-erythrocytic cycle) and thus prevent

recurrences.

Marcaine
the long-acting local anaesthetic drug
BUPIVACAINE. The effect lasts for about four hours.

Marevan
a trade name for the anticoagulant drug
WARFARIN.

Marplan
a trade name for the monoamine oxidase inhibitor
antidepression drug isocarboxazid.

Marvelon
an oral contraceptive containing the OESTROGEN
ETHINYLOESTRADIOL and the PROGESTOGEN
desogestrel.

Marzine
a trade name for the ANTIHISTAMINE and ANTI-EMETIC drug cyclizine.

Maxidex
a trade name for the steroid drug DEXAMETHASONE in the form of eyedrops.

Maxolon
a trade name for the anti-emetic and antinausea drug metoclopramide.

mebanazine
a monoamine oxidase inhibitor (MAOI) for treating severe depression. See ANTIDEPRESSANT DRUGS.

mebendazole
an ANTHELMINTIC drug used to get rid of roundworms, hookworms, threadworms and whipworms.

mebhydrolin
an ANTIHISTAMINE drug used to treat allergic
conditions such as allergic rhinitis and urticaria. A
trade name is Fabahistin.

meclozine
an anticholinergic drug that has an inhibitory
action on the vomiting centre of the brain and is
used to prevent motion sickness. A trade name is
Bonamine.

medazepam
a short-acting benzodiazepine sedative drug used
as a hypnotic. A trade name is Nobrium.

Medomet
a trade name for the antihypertensive drug
methyldopa.

Medrone
a trade name for the steroid drug
methylprednisolone.

medroxyprogesterone

a progestogen drug that can be taken by mouth and is used to treat menstrual disorders and the premenstrual syndrome. A trade name is Provera.

mefenamic acid

a non-steroidal pain-killing (ANALGESIC) and anti-inflammatory drug (NSAID).

Mefloquine should not be taken by pregnant women, or those trying to conceive.

mefruside

a thiazide-like diuretic drug used to treat high blood pressure and get rid of excess body fluid. A trade name is Baycaron.

melarsoprol

a combination of melarsan oxide and dimercaprol used to treat trypanosomiasis.

[S] *The drug is highly effective but must be used with caution because of sometimes dangerous side-effects including the Jarisch-Herxheimer reaction.*

Melleril
a trade name for the PHENOTHIAZINE antipsychotic drug thioridazine.

melphalan
a drug used in the treatment of polycythaemia vera, chronic leukaemia and myeloma.

meperidine
see PETHIDINE.

Meprate
a trade name for the anti-anxiety tranquillizer drug meprobamate.

Meptid
a trade name for the mild narcotic-like pain-killer meptazinol.

mequitazine

an ANTIHISTAMINE drug used to treat hay fever and perennial allergic rhinitis. A trade name is Primalan.

mercaptopurine

a drug used in combination with others in the treatment of leukaemia.

metaraminol

a sympathomimetic alpha adreno-receptor agonist drug used to treat severe allergic reactions (anaphylactic shock). A trade name is Aramine.

Metatone

a trade name for a mixture of THIAMINE and glycerophosphates.

metformin

a biguanide ANTIDIABETIC (oral hypoglycaemic) drug used in the treatment of maturity-onset diabetes. The drug may be dangerous to those with liver or kidney disease or a high alcohol intake.

methadone
a synthetic narcotic pain-killing (ANALGESIC) drug
with properties similar to those of morphine. It is
also used as a substitute for heroin in attempts to
manage addiction, but is widely abused.

methimazole
a drug used in the treatment of overactivity of the
thyroid gland. It is effective in reducing thyroid
activity.

[S] *Methimazole may cause agranulocytosis. A
sore throat is a warning symptom.*

Methoblastin
a trade name for METHOTREXATE.

methotrexate
an ANTIMETABOLITE and immunosuppressive drug
used to treat cancer and help in the treatment of
rheumatoid arthritis. It acts by interfering with the
metabolism of FOLIC ACID.

methyl cellulose
an inert and indigestible substance that has been used to bulk out meals in the hope of achieving weight loss. It is also used as a laxative and in artificial tears.

methyltestosterone
a male sex hormone drug sometimes used to treat severe itching caused by cirrhosis of the liver.

methylxanthine derivatives
drugs such as THEOPHYLLINE and AMINOPHYLLINE used in the treatment of asthma.

methysergide
an ergot (a type of fungus) derivative drug used to treat resistant cases of migraine. It is not without risk.

metoclopramide
an ANTI-EMETIC drug also useful for severe heartburn (reflux oesophagitis) in hiatus hernia.

Metox
a trade name for the ANTI-EMETIC drug
METOCLOPRAMIDE.

metrifonate
an organophosphorous cholinesterase inhibitor
drug used to kill the worms in schistosomiasis,
especially Schistosoma haematobium.

Metrolyl
a trade name for the ANTIBIOTIC drug
METRONIDAZOLE.

metronidazole
an ANTIBIOTIC drug effective against Trichomonas
vaginalis and Entamoeba histolytica as well as
many other organisms. It is especially useful in the
treatment of amoebic dysentery and amoebic liver
abscesses as well as anaerobic infections. A trade
name is Flagyl.

Metrozine
a trade name for METRONIDAZOLE.

metyrapone
a drug that interferes with the production of the hormone aldosterone and is used in the treatment of Cushing's syndrome. A trade name is Metopirone.

mexiletine
an anti-arrhythmic drug used in the treatment or prevention of severe heart irregularity arising in the lower chambers (ventricles). A trade name is Hypnovel.

miconazole
an imidazole antifungal drug. It can be taken by mouth or given by intravenous injection in severe systemic fungus infections.

Microgynon
a low-dose oral contraceptive pill containing ETHINYLOESTRADIOL and levonorgestrel.

KEY

The symbol [O] indicates that the drug is either available over-the-counter or that an over-the-counter drug with the same active ingredient or ingredients is available.

The symbol [»] indicates the forms in which the drug can be taken.

The symbol [S] sets out side-effects.

The symbol [W] indicates a drug recently withdrawn. These drugs should not be used.

Micronor

a low-dose oral contraceptive containing NORETHISTERONE.

Microvar

a low-dose oral contraceptive containing the progestogen drug levonorgestrel.

Midamor
a trade name for the potassium-sparing DIURETIC drug amiloride.

mifepristone (RU486)
a drug known as the 'abortion pill' that acts by blocking the action of progesterone which is essential to maintain pregnancy. A second drug, one of the prostaglandins, has to be taken within forty-eight hours to complete the expulsion of the fertilized egg. The method is said to be 95 per cent effective.

Migral, Migril
trade names for a mixture of the antimigraine drugs ERGOTAMINE, CAFFEINE and cyclizine.

Migranol
a trade name for a mixture of PARACETAMOL, ATROPINE, PAPAVERINE and nicotinic acid.

Minihep
a trade name for the anticoagulant drug HEPARIN.

Minocin
a trade name for the tetracycline ANTIBIOTIC drug
minocycline.

minoxidil
a VASODILATOR drug used in the treatment of high
blood pressure (hypertension). The drug has
acquired a barely-sustainable reputation as a hair-
restorer.

Mintezol
a trade name for THIABENDAZOLE.

misoprostol
a prostaglandin E1 drug used in the prevention and
treatment of peptic ulcer caused by NSAIDs. Trade
names: Cytotec, Napratec.

mithramycin
a drug that reduces bone metabolism and can be
useful in the treatment of Paget's disease and
hypercalcaemia.

Mixtard
a trade name for a preparation of INSULIN with a prolonged action.

Mobilan
a trade name for the non-steroidal anti-inflammatory drug (NSAID) INDOMETHACIN.

moclobemide
a new ANTIDEPRESSANT DRUG of a class known as reversible inhibitors of monoamine oxidase type A. Existing monoamine oxidase inhibitors can cause severe reactions when cheese or other tyramine-containing foods are eaten by patients taking them. These effects are less likely with reversible inhibitors.

Modecate
fluphenazine decanoate, a phenothiazine antipsychotic drug used as a depot injection for the maintenance treatment of schizophrenia and other psychotic disorders.

Moduretic
a potassium-sparing thiazide diuretic drug. See amiloride.

Mogadon
a trade name for the benzodiazepine hypnotic drug NITRAZEPAM.

Monistat
a trade name for a cream containing MICONAZOLE.

monoamine oxidase inhibitors
drugs that interfere with the action of the enzyme monoamine oxidase. This enzyme plays an important part in the breakdown of the neurotransmitters noradrenaline and 5-hydroxytryptamine (serotonin), both substances that can elevate mood. The MAO inhibitor drugs are used in the treatment of depression and anxiety.

Monophane
a trade name for an INSULIN preparation used in the control of diabetes.

Monotard

a trade name for INSULIN.

moricizine

a drug used to treat life-threatening irregularity of the heartbeat (arrhythmia). It is used only in cases in which the risks are thought to be justified.

Motillium

a trade name for the ANTI-EMETIC drug domperidone.

Motrin

a trade name for the non-steroidal anti-inflammatory drug (NSAID) IBUPROFEN.[O]

Moxacin

a trade name for AMOXICILLIN.

Mucomyst

a trade name for ACETYLCYSTEINE.

muscle-relaxant drugs

drugs, such as Curare (tubocurarine), Pancuronium,

Ballamine and Scoline (succinylcholine) used by anaesthetists to paralyse muscles and allow safer anaesthesia. In more general use are some drugs which reduce spasm of voluntary muscles without affecting voluntary movements. These may be useful in nervous system diseases, such as stroke and cerebral palsy, which cause the muscles to go into spasm, and in rheumatic and other diseases featuring painful sustained contraction of muscles. They include Lioresal (baclofen), which is a derivative of one of the body's neuro-transmitters (GABA), and Dantrium (dantrolene) which acts directly on the muscles.

Other muscle-relaxing drugs are Valium (diazepam), Trancopal (chlormezanone), Carisoma (carisoprodol) and Robaxin (methocarbamol).

Myadec
a trade name for a multivitamin and mineral preparation.

Myambutol
a trade name for ETHAMBUTOL.

Mycifradin
a trade name for NEOMYCIN.

Myciguent
a trade name for an ointment containing the ANTIBIOTIC, NEOMYCIN.

Mycostatin
a trade name for NYSTATIN.

Mydriacyl
a trade name for eye drops containing TROPICAMIDE.

Mygdalon
a trade name for the ANTI-EMETIC drug METOCLOPRAMIDE.

Mylanta
a trade name for a mixture of ALUMINIUM HYDROXIDE, MAGNESIUM HYDROXIDE and SIMETHICONE. [O]

Myleran
a trade name for BUSULPHAN.

Mynah [W]
a trade name for the antituberculosis drug
ETHAMBUTOL.

Myoquine
a trade name for QUININE.

Mysoline
a trade name for the ANTICONVULSANT drug
primidone, used in the control of epilepsy.

Mysteclin
a trade name for a mixture of the ANTIFUNGAL
drug NYSTATIN and the ANTIBIOTIC,
TETRACYCLINE.

nabilone
a cannabinoid drug, related to marijuana, used to
control severe nausea and vomiting. It is thought to
act on opiate receptors in the nervous system. A
trade name is Cesamet.

nadolol
a non-selective beta-blocker drug that acts on all
beta-adrenergic receptor sites. A trade name is
Corgard.

Nalcrom
a trade name for SODIUM CROMOGLYCATE.

nalidixic acid
a quinolone ANTIBIOTIC drug, effective against
gram negative bacilli, including Proteus species,
and much used for urinary infections. A trade name
is Negram.

nalorphine
a narcotic antagonist drug.

naloxone
a narcotic antagonist drug, chemically related to
MORPHINE, and used as an antidote to narcotic
poisoning.

naltrexone
a narcotic antagonist drug used in the treatment of

heroin and other opioid-dependent patients.

nandrolone
a male sex hormone with ANABOLIC properties.
The drug is sometimes used also to stimulate blood
cell production in aplastic anaemia. A trade name is
Durabolin.

naphazoline
an adrenergic drug that causes small blood vessels
to constrict, reducing congestion in mucous
membranes. A trade name is Antistin Privine.

[»] *It may be taken as a nasal spray.*

Naprogesic
a trade name for NAPROXEN.

Naprosyn
a trade name for NAPROXEN.

naproxen
a non-steroidal anti-inflammatory drug (NSAID). A
trade name is Naprosyn.

Narcan
a trade name for NALOXONE.

narcotic drugs
see ANALGESIC DRUGS.

Nardil
a trade name for the ANTIDEPRESSANT drug,
PHENELZINE.

Narphen
a trade name for the narcotic ANALGESIC drug
phenazocine.

Natulan
a trade name for the anticancer drug
PROCARBAZINE.

Navridex
a trade name for THIAZIDE DIURETIC drug
cyclopenthiazide.

Nazen
a trade name for NAPROXEN.

nedocromil

an anti-inflammatory drug used to treat bronchitis, bronchial asthma, late-onset asthma and exercise-induced asthma. A trade name is Tilade.

Nembudeine

a trade name for a mixture of the pain-killers PARACETAMOL and CODEINE and the sedative PENTOBARBITONE.

Nembutal

a trade name for the barbiturate sedative PENTOBARBITONE.

Neo Cortef

a trade name for a preparation, for external use, containing the anti-inflammatory drug HYDROCORTISONE and the ANTIBIOTIC, NEOMYCIN.

Neo-Hycor

a trade name for eye preparations containing the anti-inflammatory drug HYDROCORTISONE and the ANTIBIOTIC, NEOMYCIN.

Neo-Medrol
a trade name for a skin preparation containing the
steroid drug methylprednisolone and the
ANTIBIOTIC, NEOMYCIN.

Neo-Mercazole
a trade name for CARBIMAZOLE.

neomycin
an aminoglycoside ANTIBIOTIC drug derived from a
strain of Streptomyces fradiae.

[»] *Neomycin can be given by mouth to destroy
organisms in the bowel or can be used in solution
to irrigate the bladder. It is poorly absorbed into
the bloodstream. It is much too toxic to be given
by injection and can have seriously damaging
effects on hearing and on the kidneys. The drug is
widely used as a surface application in ointments.*

Neophryn
a trade name for PHENYLEPHRINE.

Neoplatin
a trade name for ciplastin, a CYTOTOXIC drug.

neostigmine
an anticholinesterase drug used in the treatment of
myasthenia gravis and to stimulate bowel and
bladder action after surgery.

Nepenthe [W]
a trade name for morphine.

Nephril
a trade name for the thiazide DIURETIC drug
polythiazide.

Netilin
a trade name for the ANTIBIOTIC netilmicin.

Neuroremed
a trade name for TRYPTOPHAN.

niacin
one of the B group of vitamins. Nicotinic acid.
Niacin is present in foods such as liver and other

meat, grains and legumes. It is a constituent of coenzymes involved in oxidation-reduction reactions in the body. Deficiency of niacin causes pellagra. Niacin is being used in the treatment of high blood cholesterol levels.

nicardipine

a calcium antagonist drug used to treat long-term stable angina pectoris. A trade name is Cardene.

niclosamide

an anthelmintic drug used to remove tapeworms. Unlike earlier treatments, it is free from side-effects. A trade name is Yomesan.

Nicorette

a nicotine preparation administered in chewing gum to help reduce the smoking habit. Nicotine is also available in skin patches for transdermal administration. Trade name Nicotinell. [O]

nicotinamide

a compound derived from nicotinic acid, see NIACIN.

nicotinic acid
see NIACIN.

Nidazol
a trade name for METRONIDAZOLE.

nifepidine
a drug used to control the symptoms of angina pectoris. It has a powerful effect in widening (dilating) arteries, including the coronary arteries, and this improves the blood supply to the heart muscle. It is often used in combination with a BETA-BLOCKER.

[S] *The drug causes flushing, headache, skin itching and dizziness.*

nifurtimox
a drug used in the treatment of South American trypanosomiasis (Chagas' disease). The drug is effective against the causal agent Trypanosoma cruzi.

[S] *Its use is associated with side-effects such as*

*nausea, vomiting, loss of appetite, abdominal pain,
muscle and joint aches, headache and vertigo.*

nikethamide
an ANALEPTIC drug used in the treatment of light
coma, drowsiness and inadequate depth of
respiration. It can raise the level of consciousness in
comatose patients so that they can be encouraged
to cough and bring up bronchial secretions.

Nilstat
a trade name for the antifungal drug NYSTATIN.

niridazole
a drug used in the treatment of schistosomiasis. It is
highly effective against the Haematobium variety
but because of its side-effects it has been largely
replaced by other drugs such as PRAZIQUANTEL.

Nitradisc
a trade name for a preparation of the angina-
relieving drug GLYCERYL TRINITRATE.

Nitrados
a trade name for NITRAZEPAM.

nitrate and nitrite drugs
drugs that relax the smooth muscle in the walls of
arteries so that they widen and more blood can
flow though. This is called vasodilatation.

The nitrates are short-term vasodilators but are
valuable in treating angina pectoris, in which the
blood supply to the heart itself is prejudiced by
narrowed coronary arteries. The nitrates are also of
value when the pumping efficiency of the heart is
reduced (heart failure).

One of the most commonly used nitrates is
nitroglycerine, the explosive, which, for medical
purposes, is mixed with inert material and made
safe. This is commonly taken in a tablet placed
under the tongue. Amyl nitrite is a volatile liquid
dispensed in thin-walled glass capsules which must
be broken before the liquid can be inhaled.
Cedocard (isosorbide dinitrate), and Elatan
(isosorbide mononitrate) are used to try to prevent

anginal attacks.

[S] *Nitrates can cause collapse by too greatly reducing the blood pressure, but this is likely only if taken in excessive dosage or if an allergic hypersensitivity has occurred.*

[S] *Nitrates may cause severe headaches by stretching the pain-sensitive tissues around the brain arteries.*

nitrazepam
a long-acting BENZODIAZEPINE hypnotic drug, widely used to promote sleep in insomnia. A trade name is Mogadon.

Nitro-bid
a trade name for a preparation of the angina-relieving drug GLYCERYL TRINITRATE.

Nitrocine
a trade name for GLYCERYL TRINITRATE (NITROGLYCERINE).

KEY
The symbol [O] indicates that the drug is either available over-the-counter or that an over-the-counter drug with the same active ingredient or ingredients is available.

The symbol [»] indicates the forms in which the drug can be taken.

The symbol [S] sets out side-effects.

The symbol [W] indicates a drug recently withdrawn. These drugs should not be used.

nitrofurazone
a drug used in the treatment of sleeping sickness (African trypanosomiasis).

nitrogen mustard
a drug used in the treatment of cancer. Nitrogen mustard is an alkylating agent – a drug that substitutes an open chain hydrocarbon radical for a hydrogen atom in molecules such as the guanine molecules in DNA. It thus prevents normal cell

replication and so is useful in the treatment of cancer.

nitroglycerine
a drug widely used to relieve the symptoms of angina pectoris. It is commonly taken in a tablet allowed to dissolve under the tongue.

Nitrolate
a trade name for a preparation of the angina-relieving drug GLYCERYL TRINITRATE.

Nitrolingual
a trade name for NITROGLYCERINE.

Nitronal
a trade name for NITROGLYCERINE.

nitroprusside
a drug used in the emergency treatment of high blood pressure. Given by controlled infusion into a vein it is the most effective known means of reducing dangerously high pressure. It must, however, be used with great care and its effects

closely monitored.

Nivaquine
a trade name for CHLOROQUINE.

Nizoral
a trade name for KETOCONAZOLE.

Nobrium
a trade name for MEDAZEPAM.

Nolvadex
a trade name for TAMOXIFEN.

non-steroidal anti-inflammatory drugs
see ANALGESIC DRUGS.

noradrenaline
an important adrenergic neuro-transmitter
released by postganglionic adrenergic nerve
endings and secreted by the inner zone (medulla)
of the adrenal gland. Noradrenaline acts chiefly on
alpha-adrenergic receptors and causes constriction
of arteries and a rise in the blood pressure. One of

the catecholamines.

norethandrolone
a synthetic ANABOLIC STEROID similar in chemical
structure to testosterone.

norethisterone
a progestogen drug commonly used alone, or in
combination with an oestrogen, as an oral
contraceptive. A trade name is Gynovlar.

Norflex
a trade name for ORPHENADRINE.

Norgesic
a trade name for ORPHENADRINE.

Normison
a trade name for TEMAZEPAM.

Nortap
a trade name for NORTRIPTYLINE.

nortriptyline
a tricyclic ANTIDEPRESSANT DRUG. A trade name is
Aventyl.

Norval
a trade name for the ANTIDEPRESSANT DRUG
myaserin.

novobiocin
an ANTIBIOTIC drug formerly of importance in the
treatment of infections with staphylococci resistant
to other antibiotics but now largely replaced by
beta-lactamase resistant penicillins.

Novocain
a trade name for the local anaesthetic drug
procaine hydrochloride.

Nozinan
a trade name for the antipsychotic drug
methotrimeprazine.

NSAIDs
non-steroidal anti-inflammatory drugs. This is a

range of drugs with pain-killing and inflammation-reducing properties that includes aspirin, aloxiprin (Palaprin forte), benorylate (Benoral), diflunisal (Dolobid), mefenamic acid (Ponstan), fenbufen (Lederfen), fenoprofen (Progesic), ibuprofen (Brufen), naproxen (Naprosyn), diclofenac (Voltarol), tolmetin (Tolectin), indomethacin (Indocid), phenylbutazone (Butazolidin) and piroxicam (Feldene).

Nubain
a trade name for the narcotic ANALGESIC nalbuphine.

Nuelin
a trade name for THEOPHYLLINE.

Nulacin
a trade name for a mixture of calcium carbonate and magnesium trisilicate. An antacid preparation.

Nupercaine
a trade name for the local anaesthetic drug CINCHOCAINE.

Nurophen
a trade name for IBUPROFEN. [O]

Nyspes
a trade name for NYSTATIN.

Nystan
a trade name for NYSTATIN.

nystatin
a drug used in the treatment of fungus infections, such as thrush (candidiasis). Nystatin is useful for external infections only as it is not absorbed when given by mouth and is too toxic to be given by injection.

Ocusert
a trade name for a device that leaches PILOCARPINE into the conjunctival sac, for the treatment of glaucoma.

oestrogens
a group of steroid sex hormones secreted mainly by the ovaries, but also by the testicles. Oestrogens

bring about the development of the female secondary sexual characteristics and act on the lining of the uterus, in conjunction with progesterone, to prepare it for implantation of the fertilized ovum.

They have some anabolic properties. Oestrogens are used to treat ovarian insufficiency and menopausal symptoms, to limit postmenopausal osteoporosis, to stop milk production (lactation) and to treat widespread cancers of the prostate gland. They are extensively used as oral contraceptives.

ofloxacin

a quinolone antibiotic drug used to treat urinary tract and sexually-acquired infections.

[»] *It is taken by mouth or given by injection.*

[S] *Possible side-effects include nausea, vomiting, skin rashes, nervous system disturbances and convulsions.*

A trade name is Tarivid.

olsalazine
a salicylate preparation used to treat mild
ulcerative colitis. A trade name is Dipentum.

omeprazole
the first of a new class of proton pump inhibitor
drugs used to control the production of stomach
acid and treat stomach and duodenal ulcers and
especially the Zollinger-Ellison syndrome.

Omeprazole can be effective in cases that have
failed to respond to H_2 receptor blocker drugs such
as ranitidine. The drug is long-acting and need only
be taken once a day. A trade name is Losec.

Omnopon-scopolamine [W]
a trade name for HYOSCINE and PAPAVERETUM.

ondansetron
a drug used for the control of severe nausea and
vomiting. Ondansetron works by opposing the
action of the neuro-transmitter serotonin.

KEY

The symbol [O] indicates that the drug is either available over-the-counter or that an over-the-counter drug with the same active ingredient or ingredients is available.

The symbol [»] indicates the forms in which the drug can be taken.

The symbol [S] sets out side-effects.

The symbol [W] indicates a drug recently withdrawn. These drugs should not be used.

Opilon

a trade name for THYMOXAMINE.

Opticrom

a trade name for SODIUM CROMOGLYCATE. [O]

Orabet

a trade name for antidiabetic drug, metformin.

Oradexon
a trade name for DEXAMETHASONE.

oral contraceptive
a drug or combination of drugs taken by women
for the purpose of preventing pregnancy. They
contain oestrogens and/or progestogens and act by
preventing the ovaries from producing eggs (ova).
They also have some effect in making the lining of
the womb less suitable for implantation of the
ovum and may make the mucus in the canal of the
cervix less easily passable by sperms. After
sterilization, oral contraceptives are the most
effective way of avoiding pregnancy. Also known
as 'the Pill'.

oral hypoglycaemic drug
one of the group of drugs used in the treatment of
maturity-onset diabetes (Type II diabetes). They
include the sulphonylurea group such as
chlorpropamide, glibenclamide, glipizide,
tolazamide and tolbutamide and the drug
metformin.

Orap
a trade name for the antipsychotic and movement disorder drug pimozide.

Orbenin
a trade name for CLOXACILLIN.

Oroxine
a trade name for the thyroid hormone THYROXINE.

orphenadrine
a drug used to relieve muscle spasm, especially in Parkinson's disease. A trade name is Disipal.

Orudis
a trade name for KETOPROFEN.

Otrivine
a trade name for the decongestant drug XYLOMETAZOLINE.

oxamniquine
a drug used in the treatment of schistosomiasis.

oxantel

a drug used to treat Trichuris worm infections.

oxatomide

an ANTIHISTAMINE drug used to treat hay fever. A trade name is Tinset.

oxazepam

a BENZODIAZEPINE tranquillizing drug. A trade name is Serenid.

oxprenolol

a beta-blocker drug used to treat angina pectoris, high blood pressure (hypertension) and disorders of heart rhythm. A trade name is Trasicor.

oxymetazoline

a sympathomimetic drug used to treat nasal congestion. A trade name is Afrazine.

oxymetholone

an anabolic steroid drug with similar actions to testosterone.

Oxymycin
a trade name for OXYTETRACYCLINE.

oxyphenbutazone
a non-steroidal anti-inflammatory drug limited to external use in ointment form. A trade name is Tanderil.

oxytetracycline
a broad-spectrum tetracycline ANTIBIOTIC derived from the mould Streptomyces rimosus. The drug is effective against a range of gram positive and gram negative organisms including Rickettsiae. A trade name is Terramycin.

oxytocic drugs
drugs that stimulate the contraction of the womb and tend to hasten childbirth. They may also be used to cause the womb to contract down after delivery of the placenta.

oxytocin
an OXYTOCIC hormone produced by the pituitary gland.

Pacitron
a trade name for the ANTIDEPRESSANT DRUG
tryptophan.

Painstop
a trade name for a mixture of the pain-killer drugs
PARACETAMOL and CODEINE. [O]

Paladac
a trade name for a preparation of VITAMINS.

Paldesic
a trade name for PARACETAMOL. [O]

Palfium
a trade name for the narcotic ANALGESIC drug
dextromoramide.

Paludrine
a trade name for the antimalarial drug proguanil.

Pamergan
a trade name for a mixture of PETHIDINE and
PROMETHAZINE.

Pameton

a trade name for a mixture of PARACETAMOL and its antidote methionine.

Pamine

a trade name for HYOSCINE.

Panadeine

a trade name for a mixture of PARACETAMOL and CODEINE. [O]

Panadol

a trade name for PARACETAMOL. [O]

Panamax

a trade name for the pain-killing drug PARACETAMOL. [O]

Panasorb

a trade name for a readily absorbable form of PARACETAMOL. [O]

Pancrease

a trade name for PANCREATIN.

Pancreatin
a preparation of pancreatic digestive enzymes that
can be taken by mouth.

Pancrex
a trade name for PANCREATIN.

Panoxyl
a trade name for BENZOYL PEROXIDE.

Pantheline
a trade name for PROPANTHELINE.

pantothenic acid
one of the B group of vitamins and a constituent of
coenzyme A which has a central role in energy
metabolism. Deficiency is rare.

papain
a mixture of enzymes found in pawpaws. Papain
includes the protein-splitting enzyme chymopapain
and this makes it useful for breaking down organic
debris and so cleaning up wounds and ulcers.
Chymopapain is used to break down material

extruded from the pulpy nuclei of intervertebral
discs (chemonucleolysis).

papaveretum
a mixture of purified opium alkaloids. Papaveretum
is mainly used for surgical premedication. Also
known as Omnopon.

papaverine
an opium derivative used as a smooth muscle
relaxant and to treat heart irregularities following
a heart attack. A trade name is Brovon.

paracetamol
an ANALGESIC drug used to treat minor pain and
to reduce fever. A trade name is Panadol. [O]

Paradex
a trade name for a mixture of
DEXTROPROPOXYPHENE and PARACETAMOL.

paraldehyde
a rapidly acting drug used by injection to control
severe excitement, delirium, mania or convulsions.

Paralgin
a trade name for PARACETAMOL. [O]

Paraspen
a trade name for the pain-killer PARACETAMOL. [O]

Parfenac [W]
a trade name for bufexamac, a drug used to relieve skin irritation.

Parlodel
a trade name for BROMOCRIPTINE.

Parmid
a trade name for METOCLOPRAMIDE.

Parmol
a trade name for the pain-killer PARACETAMOL.
[O]

Parnate
a trade name for the monamine oxidase inhibitor ANTIDEPRESSANT DRUG TRANYLCYPROMINE.

Parstelin
a trade name for a mixture of TRANYLCYPROMINE and TRIFLUOPERAZINE.

Paxadon
a trade name for pyridoxine (vitamin B6).

Paxane
a trade name for FLURAZEPAM.

Paxofen
a trade name for IBUPROFEN. [O]

pemoline
a weak stimulant of the nervous system used to threat the hyperkinetic syndrome in children. A trade name is Volital.

Penbritin
a trade name for AMPICILLIN.

Pendramine
a trade name for PENICILLAMINE.

penicillamine

a drug used to treat severe rheumatoid arthritis not responding to nonsteroidal anti-inflammatory drugs (NSAIDs).

penicillins

an important group of ANTIBIOTIC drugs. The original natural penicillin was derived from the mould Penicillium notatum but the extensive range of penicillins in use nowadays is produced synthetically.

pentaerythitol tetranitrate

a drug used to relieve the symptoms of angina pectoris. A trade name is Mycardol.

Pentalgin

a trade name for a mixture of PARACETAMOL, CODEINE and PENTOBARBITONE.

pentamidine

a drug effective against single-celled organisms (protozoa) and used in the treatment of pneumocystis carinii pneumonia in AIDS,

trypanosomiasis and kala-azar. Trade names:
Pentam 300, Nebupent.

pentazocine
a synthetic pain-killing drug which has actions
which are similar to those of MORPHINE. A trade
name is Fortral.

pentobarbitone
a now little-used barbiturate sedative and
HYPNOTIC drug of medium duration of action.
Pentobarbitone is occasionally given as a
premedication before surgery. A trade name is
Nembutal.

Pentothal
a trade name for the rapid-acting barbiturate drug
sodium thiopentone. Pentothal is commonly used
to induce general anaesthesia.

Peptard
a trade name for HYOSCYAMINE.

Percutol
a trade name for NITROGLYCERINE in a formulation for absorption through the skin.

pergolide
a dopamine agonist drug used to help in the management of Parkinsonism. A trade name is Celance.

Periactin
a trade name for the ANTIHISTAMINE and appetite-stimulating drug cyproheptadine.

Pernivit
a trade name for a mixture of NICOTINIC ACID and acetomenaphthone, used to treat chilblains.

perphenazine
a phenothiazine derivative drug used in the treatment of schizophrenia and other psychotic conditions. It is also used to relieve severe vomiting and control persistent hiccups. A trade name is Fentazin.

Persantin
a trade name for the antiplatelet drug
DIPYRIDAMOLE, used to prevent thrombosis.

Pertofran
a trade name for the tricyclic ANTIDEPRESSANT
DRUG desipramine.

pethidine
a synthetic narcotic pain-killing drug somewhat less
powerful than morphine. Pethidine is widely used
during childbirth and as a premedication.

Overuse may lead to addiction.

Pevaril
a trade name for the antifungal drug ECONAZOLE.

Phazyme
a trade name for the silicone preparation
dimethicone, used to treat indigestion from
intestinal gas. [O]

phencyclidine
a drug of abuse, commonly known as ANGEL DUST.
Also known as PCP.

phenelzine
an ANTIDEPRESSANT DRUG of the monoamine
oxidase inhibitor group. A trade name is Nardil.

Phenergan
a trade name for PROMETHAZINE.

phenformin
an oral hypoglycaemic agent formerly used in the
control of maturity onset (Type II) diabetes but now
withdrawn because of side-effects.

phenindamine
an ANTIHISTAMINE drug used to treat allergic
conditions. A trade name is Thephorin.

phenindione
an anticoagulant drug that can be taken by mouth.
Now little used because of allergic side-effects. A
trade name is Dindevan.

pheniramine

an ANTIHISTAMINE drug used to control allergic reactions. A trade name is Daneral.

phenobarbitone

a BARBITURATE drug now used mainly as an ANTICONVULSANT. Phenobarbitone is no longer used as a sedative or HYPNOTIC. A trade name is Luminal.

phenothiazine drugs

an important group of drugs widely used to treat serious mental (psychotic) illness and to relieve severe nausea and vomiting. Examples are chlorpromazine (Largactil), thioridazine (Melleril) and perphenazine (Fentanyl).

phenoxybenzamine

an alpha-adrenergic blocker drug with a powerful and persistent action, used to treat bladder neck obstruction and the effects of the adrenaline-producing tumour, the phaeochromocytoma. A trade name is Dibenyline.

phenoxymethylpenicillin
a synthetic PENICILLIN. A trade name is
Crystapen V.

Phensedyl [W]
a trade name for a mixture of CODEINE,
EPHEDRINE and PROMETHAZINE.

phentermine
a drug with an AMPHETAMINE-like action used for
appetite control in obesity. A trade name is
Duromine.

phentolamine
a drug used in the treatment of
phaeochromocytoma.

phenylbutazone
a non-steroidal anti-inflammatory drug (NSAID)
once widely used but now withdrawn from general
prescription because of its tendency to cause heart
failure from fluid retention and severe blood
disorders. It is still used, under specialist
supervision, in cases of ankylosing spondylitis. A

trade name is Butazolidin.

phenylephrine
a decongestant drug commonly used to relieve the symptoms of hay fever (allergic rhinitis) and the common cold. A trade name is Hayphryn.

phenylpropanolamine
a decongestant drug used to treat the symptoms of hay fever (allergic rhinitis), sinusitis and the common cold. A trade name is Dimotapp LA. [O]

pholcodine
an opioid drug used mainly to suppress coughs. [O]

Pholcomed
a trade name for a mixture of PAPAVERINE and the cough suppressant pholcodine.

pilocarpine
a drug used in the form of eye-drops to treat glaucoma. Pilocarpine causes extreme constriction of the pupils. Trade names are Sno Pilo and Pilopt.

pimozide
a long-acting phenothiazine antipsychotic drug of
the diphenylbutylpiperidine group that is also used
in the treatment of the Gilles de la Tourette's
syndrome. A trade name is Orap.

pindolol
a BETA-BLOCKER drug used in the treatment of
angina pectoris, high blood pressure and heart
irregularity. A trade name is Visken.

piperazine
an ANTHELMINTIC drug used to paralyse
roundworms and threadworms, which are then
passed with the faeces. A trade name is Antepar.

pirenzepine
a drug used to cut secretion of acid by the stomach
in the treatment of peptic ulcer.

Piriton
a trade name for the ANTIHISTAMINE drug
CHLORPHENIRAMINE.

KEY

The symbol [O] indicates that the drug is either available over-the-counter or that an over-the-counter drug with the same active ingredient or ingredients is available.

The symbol [»] indicates the forms in which the drug can be taken.

The symbol [S] sets out side-effects.

The symbol [W] indicates a drug recently withdrawn. These drugs should not be used.

---

piroxicam

a non-steroidal anti-inflammatory drug (NSAID) used mainly to control symptoms in the various forms of arthritis. A trade name is Feldene.

Pitressin

a trade name for vasopressin, a natural body hormone used in the treatment of pituitary-originated diabetes insipidus.

pivampicillin

a broad-spectrum penicillin-type ANTIBIOTIC used to treat bronchitis, pneumonia, skin infections, urinary infections and gonorrhoea. Trade names: Pondocillin.

pivmecillinam

an amidino penicillin ANTIBIOTIC used to treat urinary infections and other infections with mecillinam-sensitive organisms. A trade name is Selexid.

pizotifen

an ANTIHISTAMINE drug used in the treatment of severe migraine. A trade name is Sanomigran.

Planequil

a trade name for the antimalarial drug hydroxychloroquine.

Platamine

a trade name for the anticancer drug cisplatin.

Platosin
a trade name for the anticancer drug cisplatin.

podophyllin
a resin that may be applied locally in the treatment of various kinds of warts. Podophyllin is damaging to normal skin and must be applied with care.

Polybactrin
a trade name for a mixture of the ANTIBIOTICS bacitracin, NEOMYCIN and polymyxin. For external use.

Polycrol
a trade name for a mixture of the antacid drugs aluminium hydroxide and magnesium hydroxide and the antifoaming agent dimethicone. [O]

polymyxins
a group of five polypeptide ANTIBIOTIC drugs active against various gram negative bacteria. They are used almost exclusively as external applications in ointments and eye and ear drops because of their toxicity if taken internally.

Polytar
a trade name for COAL TAR. [O]

Ponderax
a trade name for the weight-control drug
FENFLURAMINE.

Ponstan
a trade name for the non-steroidal anti-
inflammatory drug MEFENAMIC ACID.

potassium channel blocker
a drug that closes the channels in cell membranes
through which potassium ions pass out of cells. The
effect of this is to increase the excitability and
probability of action of the cells. Potassium channel
blockers include the sulphonylurea group of drugs
used to treat maturity-onset diabetes. These
increase the output of INSULIN from the beta cells
of the Islets of Langerhans in the pancreas.

potassium channel opener
a drug that opens the channels in cell membranes
through which potassium ions pass. Efflux of

potassium reduces the excitability of the cell so that it is less likely to act. Potassium channel openers include the muscle relaxant drugs minoxidil and hydralazine used to treat high blood pressure.

potassium permanganate
a soluble compound that gives a skin-staining, deep purple solution with antiseptic and astringent properties.

povidone iodine
a mild antiseptic for local application, used in many proprietary creams, ointments and washes. A trade name is Betadine. [O]

Pragmatar
a trade name for a mixture of coal tar, the skin-softening agent salicylic acid and sulphur. [O]

Pramin
a trade name for metoclopramide.

Praminil
a trade name for IMIPRAMINE.

pravastatin
see HMG CoA reductase inhibitors.

Praxilene
a trade name for the VASODILATOR drug
naftidrofuryl.

praziquantel
an anthelmintic drug used to dispose of
tapeworms, schistosomes, liver flukes and lung
flukes. A trade name is Biltricide.

prazosin
a drug that widens arteries (vasodilator) and is used
in the treatment of high blood pressure, heart
failure and Raynaud's phenomenon. A trade name
is Hypovase.

Prednefrin Forte
a trade name for eye drops containing
PREDNISOLONE and PHENYLEPHRINE.

Prednesol
a trade name for PREDNISOLONE.

prednisolone
a semisynthetic CORTICOSTEROID DRUG derived from the natural steroid hormone cortisol and used in the treatment of a wide range of inflammatory disorders. A trade name is Predsol.

prednisone
a synthetic CORTICOSTEROID DRUG used to reduce inflammation and relieve symptoms in rheumatoid arthritis, ulcerative colitis and many other conditions. A trade name is Decortisyl.

Predsol
a trade name for PREDNISOLONE.

Prefil
a trade name for the bulk-forming antidiarrhoeal agent sterculia.

Pregaday
a trade name for a mixture of FOLIC ACID and iron.

Premarin
a trade name for a preparation of conjugated oestrogens. The name is said to derive from the source – pregnant mare's urine.

Prestim
a trade name for a mixture of the thiazide diuretic drug bendrofluazide and the beta-blocking drug timolol.

Priadel
a trade name for LITHIUM.

primaquine
a drug used in the treatment of Plasmodium vivax and Plasmodium ovale malaria.

primidone
an ANTICONVULSANT drug used in the treatment
of epilepsy. A trade name is Mysoline.

Primodian
a trade name for the male sex hormone
TESTOSTERONE.

Primogyn
a trade name for the female sex hormone
oestradiol.

Primolut N
a trade name for NORETHISTERONE.

Primoteston
a trade name for TESTOSTERONE.

Primperan
a trade name for the ANTI-EMETIC drug
metoclopramide.

Pripsen
a trade name for a mixture of the ANTHELMINTIC

drug PIPERAZINE and the laxative senna.

Pro-Actidil [W]
a trade name for the ANTIHISTAMINE drug
triprolidine. [O]

Pro-Banthine
a trade name for the antispasmodic drug
propantheline.

probenecid
a drug used in the treatment of gout. Probenecid
acts by increasing the rate of excretion of uric acid
in the urine and thus lowering its levels in the
body. A trade name is Benemid.

probucol
a cholesterol-lowering drug. A trade name is
Lurselle.

procainamide
a local anaesthetic-like drug used intravenously to
control heart irregularities by its action to diminish
the excitability of the conducting bundles in the

heart muscle. A trade name is Pronestyl.

procaine
a local anaesthetic drug now largely replaced by
others that are more quickly effective or of more
persistent action.

procarbazine
an anticancer drug used especially in the treatment
of lymphomas. A trade name is Natulan.

prochlorperazine
a PHENOTHIAZINE derivative antipsychotic drug
used to treat schizophrenia and mania and to
relieve nausea and vomiting. A trade name is
Stemetil.

procyclidine
an ANTICHOLINERGIC drug used to treat
Parkinson's disease. A trade name is Arpicolin.

Prodexin
a trade name for the antacid drug magnesium
carbonate.

Proflex
a trade name for IBUPROFEN. [O]

Progesic
a trade name for the non-steroidal anti-inflammatory drug (NSAID) fenoprofen.

progestogen drugs
a group of drugs chemically and pharmacologically similar to the natural hormone progesterone. They are used in oral contraceptives to alter the womb lining so that it is less receptive to a fertilized egg and to make the mucus in the cervix less readily penetrable by sperms. They are also used to treat menstrual disorders.

Progout
a trade name for ALLOPURINOL.

proguanil
an antimalarial drug mainly used for prevention (as a prophylactic). A trade name is Paludrine.

promazine
a phenothiazine derivative antipsychotic drug used as a sedative. A trade name is Sparine.

promethazine
an ANTIHISTAMINE drug used to relieve itching, to control motion sickness and as a sedative. A trade name is Phenergan.

Prominal
a trade name for the barbiturate methylphenobarbitone.

Prondol [W]
a trade name for the ANTIDEPRESSANT DRUG iprindole.

Pronestyl
a trade name for the ANTI-ARRHYTHMIC drug PROCAINAMIDE.

propantheline
an antispasmodic drug used to relieve bowel spasm and to treat the irritable bowel syndrome and

urinary incontinence caused by an irritable bladder. A trade name is Pro-Banthine.

propranolol

a beta-blocker drug used to treat high blood pressure (hypertension), angina pectoris and heart irregularities (cardiac arrhythmias). A trade name is Inderal.

propylthiouracil

a drug used to treat overactivity of the thyroid gland (hyperthyroidism).

prostaglandin drugs

synthetic prostaglandins used to induce labour or procure abortion, to treat persistent ductus arteriosus and to relieve peptic ulcer. The group include dinoprostone (prostaglandin E_2) and dinoprost (prostaglandin F_{2a})

prostaglandins

a group of unsaturated fatty acid mediators occurring throughout the tissues and body fluids. They are generated from cell membrane phospholipids by the action of phospholipase A_2 and function as hormones. They have many different actions. They cause constriction or widening of arteries, they stimulate pain nerve endings, they promote or inhibit aggregation of blood platelets and hence influence blood clotting, they induce abortion, reduce stomach acid secretion and relieve asthma. Some pain-killing drugs, such as aspirin, act by preventing the release of prostaglandins from injured tissue.

Prostigmin
a trade name for NEOSTIGMINE.

protamine zinc insulin
a slow-release form of INSULIN with an action lasting for twelve to twenty-four hours. A trade name is Humulin Zn.

Protaphane
a trade name for a form of INSULIN.

Prothezine
a trade name for PROMETHAZINE.

Prothiaden
a trade name for the tricyclic ANTIDEPRESSANT DRUG dothiepin.

prothionamide
a drug used in the treatment of tuberculosis resistant to commoner drugs.

Protran
a trade name for CHLORPROMAZINE.

protriptyline
an ANTIDEPRESSANT DRUG used especially to treat narcolepsy or depression associated with pathological lethargy. A trade name is Concordin.

Pro-Vent
a trade name for the asthma-control drug theophylline.

Provera
a trade name for the PROGESTOGEN drug methylprogesterone.

Pro-Viron
a trade name for the male sex hormone drug mesterolone.

Prozac
a trade name for fluoxetine.

pseudoephedrine
a drug with adrenaline-like actions used as a decongestant and bronchodilator. It is widely used as a constituent of proprietary cold and cough remedies. [O]

Psoradrate
a trade name for a mixture of the antipsoriasis drug dithranol and urea.

psoralen drugs
a plant derivative (coumarin) which, when applied to the skin or taken internally, increases the tendency of the skin to pigment under the action of ultraviolet light. This effect is exploited in the treatment of psoriasis and other skin conditions. See also puva.

Psorin
a trade name for a mixture of the antipsoriasis drug DITHRANOL, COAL TAR and the skin-softening agent SALICYLIC ACID.

psychedelic drugs
see HALLUCINOGENIC DRUGS.

psychotropic drugs
drugs that effect the state of the mind, including sedatives, TRANQUILLIZERS, ANTIPSYCHOTIC drugs and HALLUCINOGENIC drugs.

Pulmadil
a trade name for the bronchodilator drug rimiterol.

Pulmicort
a trade name for the CORTICOSTEROID DRUG bursonide.

Puri-Nethol
a trade name for the anticancer drug MERCAPTOPURINE.

pyrantel
an ANTHELMINTIC drug used to treat intestinal
worm infestations, especially roundworms and
threadworms.

[S] *Side-effects occur only with large doses and
include headache, dizziness, skin rash and fever.*

Trade names: Antiminth, Combantrin.

pyrazinamide
an antituberculous drug that diffuses well into the
cerebro-spinal fluid and is used to treat tuberculous
meningitis. A trade name is Rifater.

pyrazolone drugs
a group of non-steroidal anti-inflammatory drugs
(NSAIDs) that includes phenylbutazone and
azapropazone.

pyridostigmine
a nerve-stimulating Cholinergic drug that acts by
interfering with the enzyme cholinesterase that

breaks down acetylcholine. It is used in the treatment of myastenia gravis.

[»] *It is taken by mouth or given by injection.*

[S] *Possible side-effects include nausea, vomiting, diarrhoea, abdominal pain, diarrhoea, sweating and increased salivation.*

A trade name is Mestinon.

pyridoxine
one of the B_6 group of vitamins. Deficiency is rare.

pyrimethamine
a drug used in the treatment of malaria and toxoplasmosis. A trade name is Daraprim.

pyrithioxine
a vitamin B_6 derivative said to be useful in the management of senile dementia and behavioural disorders in children.

KEY

The symbol **[O]** indicates that the drug is either available over-the-counter or that an over-the-counter drug with the same active ingredient or ingredients is available.

The symbol **[»]** indicates the forms in which the drug can be taken.

The symbol **[S]** sets out side-effects.

The symbol **[W]** indicates a drug recently withdrawn. These drugs should not be used.

Pyrogastrone

a trade name for a mixture of the antacid drugs aluminium hydroxide, sodium bicarbonate and magnesium trisilicate, the antifoaming agent alginic acid and the ulcer-protective drug carbenoxolone.

qinghaosu

a Chinese herbal drug used for 2000 years to treat malaria. The active ingredient is a sesquiterpene lactone that greatly reduces the number of malarial parasites in the blood. The mode of action is not fully understood but is currently being investigated and trials of the drug have recently started in the West.

quinacrine
a yellow acridine dye useful in studying chromosomal structure because of its property of fluorescing when bound to certain regions of chromosomes. Also known as mepacrine. Quinacrine was once widely used to prevent malaria and to remove tapeworms.

Quinate
a trade name for QUININE.

Quinbisul
a trade name for QUININE.

Quinidex SA
a trade name for QUINIDINE.

quinidine
a drug derived from QUININE and used to control
irregularity or excessive rapidity of the heart beat
by depressing the excitability of the muscle.

Quinidoxin
a trade name for QUINIDINE.

quinine
the first drug found to be effective in the
prevention and treatment of MALARIA. Quinine
was originally derived from the bark of the
cinchona tree. It is still used to treat
CHLOROQUINE-resistant malaria but is no longer
used as a prophylactic.

Quinoctal
a trade name for QUININE.

quinolone drugs
a group of synthetic ANTIBIOTIC drugs that
includes nalidixic acid, oxfloxacin and enoxacin.
These drugs act by inactivating an enzyme, DNA
gyrase, necessary for replication of the organisms.

They are often useful for treating infections with organisms that have become resistant to other antibiotics. They are administered by mouth. Psychiatric disturbances occasionally occur.

Quinsul
a trade name for QUININE.

Rafen
a trade name for IBUPROFEN. [O]

ranitidine
an H_2 (histamine-2) receptor antagonist drug used to reduce acid secretion in cases of peptic ulceration. A trade name is Zantac.

Rapidard
a trade name for INSULIN.

rauwolfia
dried extracts from the plant Rauwolfia serpentina that contains the alkaloid RESERPINE, a sedative and tranquillizing drug that also lowers blood pressure.

Redoxon
a trade name for vitamin C.

Refrane
a trade name for LOBELINE.

Renitec
a trade name for ENALAPRIL.

reserpine
a RAUWOLFIA alkaloid that decreases the
concentration of the neuro-transmitter 5-
hydroxytryptamine (serotonin) in the nervous
system and has a sedative, antihypertensive and
tranquillizing effect.

Respolin
a trade name for SALBUTAMOL.

Resprim
a trade name for CO-TRIMOXAZOLE.

Retin A
a trade name for TRETINOIN.

retinoid drug
one of a group of drugs related to vitamin A that
act on the skin to cause drying and peeling and a
reduction in oil (sebum) production. These effects
can be useful in the treatment of acne, psoriasis,
ichthyosis and other skin disorders. A trade name is
Retin-A, Roaccutane.

[»]*They are administered by mouth or applied as a
cream.*

[S] *Side-effects include severe fetal abnormalities
(if taken by pregnant women), toxic effects on
babies (if taken by breast-feeding mothers), liver
and kidney damage, excessive drying, redness and
itching of the skin, and muscle pain and stiffness.*

Retrovir
an antiviral drug with some useful effect against
the retrovirus HIV that causes AIDS. Also known as
AZT (azidothymidine) and ZIDOVUDINE.

Rheumacin
a trade name for INDOMETHACIN.

ribavirin
an antiviral drug effective against a range of both
DNA and RNA viruses including the herpes group
and those causing hepatitis, several strains of
influenza and Lassa fever. Unfortunately, it
antagonizes the action of zidovudine (AZT) against
HIV. A trade name is Virazole.

riboflavin
vitamin B_2.

Rifadin
a trade name for RIFAMPICIN.

rifampicin
an ANTIBIOTIC drug used mainly to treat
tuberculosis and leprosy, but also Legionnaire's
disease, prostatitis, endocarditis and osteomyelitis.

*Rifampicin interferes with the action of oral
contraceptives.*

rimiterol
a bronchodilator drug which is used during the

treatment of asthma and bronchitis. A trade name
is Pulmadil.

Rimycin
a trade name for RIFAMPICIN.

ritodrine
a drug that relaxes the muscles of the womb and is
used to prevent the onset of premature labour. A
trade name is Yutopar.

Rivotril
a trade name for CLONAZEPAM.

Rynacrom
a trade name for SODIUM CROMOGLYCATE. [O]

Rythmodan
a trade name for DISOPYRAMIDE.

Sabin vaccine
an effective oral vaccine used to immunize against
poliomyelitis. This vaccine contains live attenuated
viruses that spread by the fecal-oral route in the

manner of the original disease, thus effectively
disseminating the protection. (Albert Bruce Sabin,
Russian-born American bacteriologist, b. 1906.)

Salazopyrin
a trade name for the drug SULPHASALAZINE used
to treat rheumatoid arthritis, ulcerative colitis and
Crohn's disease.

Salbulin
a trade name for SALBUTAMOL.

salbutamol
a bronchodilator drug used to treat asthma,
chronic bronchitis and emphysema. It is also
sometimes used to relax the muscle of the womb
and prevent premature labour.

salicylates
a group of anti-inflammatory, mildly ANALGESIC
and fever-reducing (antipyretic) drugs that includes
aspirin, sodium salicylate and BENORYLATE.

salicylic acid
a drug that softens and loosens the horny outer layer of the skin (the epidermis) and is used in the treatment of various skin disorders such as psoriasis, ichthyosis, warts and callosities. **[O]**

Salk vaccine
a killed virus antipoliomyelitis vaccine developed by American microbiologist Jonas Salk (b. 1914).

salmeterol
a beta-adrenergic agonist drug used to treat severe asthma. A trade name is Serevent.

salsalate
a non-steroidal anti-inflammatory drug (NSAID).

Saluric
a trade name for the drug CHLOROTHIAZIDE.

Sandimmun
a trade name for CYCLOSPORIN.

Sandocal
a trade name for a calcium preparation.

Scop
a trade name for HYOSCINE.

scopolamine
an ATROPINE-like drug which is used in premedication as a sedative and to dry up respiratory and salivary secretions.

Seconal
a trade name for the barbiturate drug quinalbarbitone.

Sectral
a trade name for ACEBUTOLOL.

Securon
a trade name for the drug VERAPAMIL.

sedative drugs
a group of drugs that includes ANTI-ANXIETY DRUGS, HYPNOTIC DRUGS, some ANTIPSYCHOTIC

DRUGS and some ANTIDEPRESSANT DRUGS.

selective serotonin re-uptake inhibitor drugs
drugs that prolong the complex action of the brain
neuro-transmitter serotonin (5-hydroxytryptamine).
They achieve this by preventing the normal
removal of the neuro-transmitter from synapses
between nerves.

The effect of this, which is not yet fully understood,
is to produce relief of depression and a sense of
well-being. These drugs, such as fluoxetine
(Prozac), sertraline, paroxetine and fluvoxamine,
have been described as 'happiness drugs'. They are
much less liable to produce undesirable side-effects
than other ANTIDEPRESSANT DRUGS and seem less
toxic in overdose.

*Some patients taking them have shown adverse
effects including uncharacteristically violent
behaviour. Early reports that they predispose to
suicide have not been substantiated.*

selegiline

a selective MONOAMINE OXIDASE INHIBITOR drug used in the treatment of Parkinsonism. Selegiline is thought to retard the breakdown of DOPAMINE. A trade name is Eldepryl.

selenium

a trace element recently found to be an essential component of the enzyme deiodinase which catalyses the production of triiodothyronine (T_3) from thyroxine (T_4) in the thyroid gland. Selenium deficiency prevents the formation of T_3.

selenium sulphide

a selenium compound used to treat dandruff and used as a shampoo. A trade name is Lenium, Selsun.

Selsun

a trade name for a SELENIUM-containing shampoo used to treat dandruff.

Semitard MC

a trade name for a form of INSULIN having medium duration of action.

Septrin
a trade name for the antibacterial drug CO-TRIMOXAZOLE.

Serc
a trade name for the drug betahistidine used in the treatment of Ménière's disease.

Serenace
a trade name for the tranquillizing drug HALOPERIDOL.

Serepax
a trade name for OXAZEPAM.

Serophene
a trade name for the drug clomiphene, used in the treatment of infertility.

Sigmacort
a trade name for HYDROCORTISONE. [O]

Simeco
a trade name for a mixture of ALUMINIUM

445

HYDROXIDE, MAGNESIUM HYDROXIDE and SIMETHICONE. [O]

simethicone
a silicone-based material with antifoaming properties used in the treatment of flatulence and often incorporated into antacid remedies. Simethicone is also used as a water-repellant skin protecting agent in the management of nappy rash and other skin disorders.

simvastatin
see HMG CoA reductase inhibitors.

Sinequan
a trade name for the tranquillizing drug doxepin.

Sintisone
a trade name for PREDNISOLONE.

Sinutab Antihistamine
a trade name for a mixture of PARACETAMOL, PSEUDOEPHEDRINE and CHLORPHENIRAMINE.

Sinuzets
a trade name for capsules containing
PARACETAMOL, PSEUDOEPHEDRINE and
PHENYLEPHRINE. [O]

Skitz
a trade name for BENZOYL PEROXIDE.

sleeping drugs
a group of drugs used to promote sleep. The group
includes many BENZODIAZEPINE drugs, some
ANTIHISTAMINE DRUGS, ANTIDEPRESSANT DRUGS
and chloral hydrate. The BARBITURATE drugs, once
widely used for this purpose, have fallen into
disrepute. The same now seems to be happening to
the benzodiazepines.

Slo-Bid
a trade name for THEOPHYLLINE.

Slo-Fe
a trade name for an IRON preparation.

Slow-K
a trade name for a POTASSIUM preparation.

sodium aurothiomalate
a gold preparation given by injection for the
treatment of rheumatoid arthritis.

sodium bicarbonate
baking soda. An antacid drug used to relieve
indigestion, heartburn and the pain of peptic ulcer.
Sodium bicarbonate is not a preferred antacid as it
leads to the production of carbon dioxide and
'rebound' acid production.

sodium cromoglycate
a drug used to treat hay fever (allergic rhinitis),
allergic conjunctivitis, food allergy and allergic
asthma. Cromoglycate stabilizes the mast cell
membrane and prevents the release of histamine.

sodium pentothal
a rapid-acting BARBITURATE drug used for the
induction of general anaesthesia.

sodium salicylate
an ANALGESIC drug used to treat rheumatic fever.
It has no advantages over ASPIRIN (acetyl salicylic
acid) and the same adverse effects.

sodium valproate
an anticonvulsant drug used to treat epilepsy.

Sofradex
a trade name for eye or ear drops or ointment
containing DEXAMETHASONE, FRAMYCETIN and
GRAMICIDIN.

Soframycin
a trade name for the ANTIBIOTIC drug
FRAMYCETIN.

Solcode
a trade name for a mixture of ASPIRIN and
CODEINE. [O]

Solone
a trade name for PREDNISOLONE.

Solprin
a trade name for ASPIRIN.

Solu-Cortef
a trade name for HYDROCORTISONE. [O]

Solu-Medrol
a trade name for METHYLPREDNISOLONE.

somatrem
a preparation of human growth hormone used to treat short stature caused by growth hormone deficiency.

Sominex
a trade name for the ANTIHISTAMINE drug PROMETHAZINE used as a sedative.

Somophyllin
a trade name for AMINOPHYLLINE.

Sone
a trade name for PREDNISONE.

Soneryl
a trade name for the barbiturate drug
BUTOBARBITONE.

sorbitol
a sweetening agent derived from glucose.

sotalol
a long-acting beta-blocker drug used to treat
irregularity of the heart action. A trade name is
Beta-Cardone.

Span K
a trade name for a POTASSIUM preparation.

Spanish fly
dried extract of the blister beetle, Lytta vesicatoria.
Cantharides. This is a highly irritating and
poisonous substance with an unjustified reputation
as an aphrodisiac

Sparine
a trade name for the phenothiazine antipsychotic
drug promazine.

KEY

The symbol [O] indicates that the drug is either available over-the-counter or that an over-the-counter drug with the same active ingredient or ingredients is available.

The symbol [»] indicates the forms in which the drug can be taken.

The symbol [S] sets out side-effects.

The symbol [W] indicates a drug recently withdrawn. These drugs should not be used.

Spiretic

a trade name for the potassium-sparing diuretic SPIRONOLACTONE.

spironolactone

a DIURETIC drug that does not lead to loss of potassium from the body. It is an antagonist of the hormone aldosterone. A trade name is Aldactone.

Stafoxil
a trade name for the ANTIBIOTIC FLUCLOXACILLIN.

stanozolol
an anabolic steroid drug used to treat the effects of
deep vein thrombosis and systemic sclerosis. A
trade name is Stromba.

Staphlipen
a trade name for the ANTIBIOTIC FLUCLOXACILLIN.

Staphylex
a trade name for FLUCLOXACILLIN.

Stelazine
a trade name for the phenothiazine antipsychotic
drug and ANTI-EMETIC trifluoperazine.

Stemetil
a trade name for the phenothiazine antipsychotic
drug and ANTI-EMETIC prochlorperazine.

steroid
any member of the class of fat-soluble organic

compounds based on a structure of seventeen carbon atoms arranged in three connected rings of six, six and five carbons. The steroids include the adrenal cortex hormones, the sex hormones, progestogens, bile salts, sterols and a wide range of synthetic compounds produced for therapeutic purposes. The natural steroid hydrocortisone is also in widespread use as a drug. Anabolic steroids are male sex hormones that stimulate the production of protein.

stilboestrol
a synthetic oestrogen drug similar in action to the natural hormone oestradiol. Stilboestrol is used to treat cancer of the prostate, some types of breast cancer and postmenopausal atrophic vaginitis. A trade name is Tampovagan.

Streptase
a trade name for the blood clot dissolving enzyme drug STREPTOKINASE.

streptokinase
protein-splitting enzyme used as a drug to dissolve

blood clot in a coronary artery so as to minimize the degree of myocardial infarction during a heart attack. It is also used to treat pulmonary embolism.

streptomycin
an aminoglycoside ANTIBIOTIC drug used to treat some rare infections such as brucellosis, glanders, plague, tuberculosis and tularaemia.

[S] *It is avoided for commoner infections because of its side-effects, which include deafness and tinnitus.*

strychnine
a bitter-tasting, highly poisonous substance occurring in the seeds of Strychnos species of tropical trees and shrubs. Poisoning causes restlessness, stiffness of the face and neck, exaggerated sensations, extreme arching of the back (opisthotonus) and death from paralysis of breathing unless artificial ventilation is used.

sucralfate
an aluminium-containing drug that forms a

protective coating over the stomach or duodenal lining. Sucralfate is used in the treatment of peptic ulcer.

[S] *A fairly common side-effect is constipation.*

A trade name is Antepsin.

Sudafed
a trade name for PSEUDOEPHEDRINE. **[O]**

sulfadoxine
a SULPHONAMIDE DRUG used as an adjunct to CHLOROQUINE in the treatment of Falciparum malaria. A trade name is Fansidar.

sulindac
a non-steroidal anti-inflammatory drug (NSAID). A trade name is Clinoril.

sulphacetamide
a SULPHONAMIDE DRUG limited to external use, as in eye drops for the treatment of conjunctivitis. A trade name is Albucid.

sulphadiazine
a readily absorbed and quickly eliminated
SULPHONAMIDE DRUG used in mixtures with other
similar drugs in the treatment of various infections,
especially urinary infections. A trade name is
Sulphatriad.

sulphasalazine
a compound of a SULPHONAMIDE DRUG and 5-
aminosalicylic acid used to treat rheumatoid
arthritis, ulcerative colitis and Crohn's disease. A
trade name is Salazopyrin.

sulphinpyrazone
a uricosuric drug used to reduce the frequency of
attacks of gout. A trade name is Anturan.

sulphonamide drugs
a large group of antibacterial drugs now largely
superseded by the ANTIBIOTICS except for the
treatment of urinary tract infections. The group
includes SULFADOXINE, SULPHACETAMIDE,
SULPHADIAZINE, sulphadimethoxine,
sulphadimidine, sulphamerazine, sulphamethazine,

sulphamethizole, sulphamethoxazole and sulfathiazole.

sulphonylureas
a class of drugs used in the treatment of maturity onset (Type II), non-insulin dependency diabetes. They are taken by mouth. Also known as oral hypoglycaemic drugs.

sulpiride
an antipsychotic drug. A trade name is Dolmatil.

Sulpitil
a trade name for the antipsychotic drug SULPIRIDE.

sumatriptan
a sterotonin antagonist drug that has been found effective in the symptomatic treatment of acute migraine.

[»] *It is taken by mouth or given by injection.*

[S] *Possible side-effects include nausea, vomiting,*

skin rashes, nervous system disturbances and convulsions.

A trade name is Imigran.

Supradyn
a trade name for a multivitamin and mineral preparation.

suramin
a drug used in the treatment of trypanosomiasis.

Surem
a trade name for the benzodiazepine drug NITRAZEPAM.

surfactant
a substance that reduces surface tension and promotes wetting of surfaces. The lungs contain a surfactant to prevent collapse of the alveoli.

Surmontil
a trade name for the tricyclic ANTIDEPRESSANT DRUG TRIMIPRAMINE.

Suscard

a trade name for the artery-dilating drug
GLYCERYL TRINITRATE (nitroglycerine).

Sustac

a trade name for the artery-dilating drug
GLYCERYL TRINITRATE (nitroglycerine).

Sustamycin

a trade name for the ANTIBIOTIC TETRACYCLINE.

Sustanon

a trade name for the male sex hormone drug
TESTOSTERONE.

sympathomimetic drugs

drugs which act on the body in such a way as to
cause effects similar to those of the sympathetic
part of the autonomic nervous system – generally
stimulating effects, with an increase in the heart
rate, an increase in the blood supply to the
voluntary muscles, a slowing of digestion,
dilatation of the pupils, widening of the lung air
tubes (bronchial tubes) and tightening of

sphincters. This effect is produced by the natural hormones adrenaline and noradrenaline and by drugs such as amphetamine, ephedrine, isoprenaline, methoxamine, salbutamol, phenylephrine, metaproterenol, terbutaline and soterenol.

The effect of sympathomimetic drugs is complicated by the fact that there are several different receptors for adrenaline-like substances. These are divided into the alpha-adrenergic receptors (alpha-1 and alpha-2) and the beta-adrenergic receptors (beta-1 and beta-2). Some drugs stimulate some of these receptors, but not others; some stimulate all adrenoreceptors.

Drugs which block the adrenoreceptors are, in general, antagonistic to the sympathomimetic drugs.

Synadrin
a trade name for the CALCIUM CHANNEL BLOCKER drug prenylamine.

KEY

The symbol [O] indicates that the drug is either available over-the-counter or that an over-the-counter drug with the same active ingredient or ingredients is available.

The symbol [»] indicates the forms in which the drug can be taken.

The symbol [S] sets out side-effects.

The symbol [W] indicates a drug recently withdrawn. These drugs should not be used.

Synalar
a trade name for the steroid drug fluocinolone, used for local applications.

Synandone
a trade name for the steroid drug fluocinolone, used for local applications.

Synflex
a trade name for the non-steroidal anti-

inflammatory drug (NSAID) NAPROXEN.

Synopessin
a trade name for the drug lypressin used in the treatment of diabetes insipidus.

Syntaris
a trade name for the CORTICOSTEROID DRUG flunisolide.

Syntocinon
a trade name for the womb muscle stimulating drug OXYTOCIN.

Syraprim
a trade name for the antibacterial drug trimethoprim.

Sytron
a trade name for the iron preparation, sodium iron edetate, used in the treatment of anaemia.

Tagamet
a trade name for CIMETIDINE.

talampicillin

a penicillin type ANTIBIOTIC of the ampicillin ester class, effective against Gram's stain positive and many Gram negative organisms. Talampicillin achieves higher blood concentrations than ampicillin. A trade name is Talpen.

Talpen [W]

a trade name for the penicillin ANTIBIOTIC talampicillin.

Tamofen

a trade name for TAMOXIFEN.

tamoxifen

a drug that blocks oestrogen receptors and is useful in the treatment of certain cancers, especially breast cancer. It also stimulates egg production from the ovaries and can be used to treat infertility. A trade name is Tamofen.

Tanderil [W]

a trade name for an eye ointment containing oxyphenbutazone.

taxol

an anticancer drug which was formerly obtainable only from the bark of the Pacific yew tree but now synthesized. It has also been produced by biotechnological plant tissue culture methods. Taxol interacts with tubulin, a protein involved in cell division and has been found to exercise control on the growth of ovarian, breast and lung cancers. Its use remains experimental.

Tegretol

a trade name for CARBAMAZEPINE.

Teldane

a trade name for TERFENADINE.

Temaze

a trade name for TEMAZEPAM.

temazepam

a benzodiazepine drug used to treat insomnia. A trade name is Normison.

Temgesic
a trade name for BUPRENORPHINE.

Tempra
a trade name for PARACETAMOL. [O]

Tenopt
a trade name for eye drops containing TIMOLOL.

Tenormin
a trade name for ATENOLOL.

Tensium
a trade name for DIAZEPAM.

Tenuate dospan
a trade name for the appetite-reducing drug
DIETHYLPROPION.

terbinafine
This is used to help to control bleeding from
varicose veins of the gullet (oesophageal varices) by
constricting the small arteries in the intestinal tract.

terbutaline
a bronchodilator drug used in the treatment of
asthma, bronchitis and emphysema. It is also used
to relax the muscle of the womb and prevent
premature labour. A trade name is Bricanyl.

terfenadine
an antihistamine drug used to treat allergic rhinitis
and urticaria.

[»] *It is taken by mouth.*

[S] *Possible side-effects include headache,*
digestive upset, skin rashes, sweating, heart
irregularity.

A trade name is Triludan.

terlipressin
a drug that releases vasopressin over a period of
hours. This is used to help to control bleeding from
oesophageal varices by constricting the small
arteries in the intestinal tract.

terodiline

a drug used to treat heart irregularity but
withdrawn in 1991 because of adverse reactions.

Terramycin

a trade name for the tetracycline ANTIBIOTIC
OXYTETRACYCLINE.

Testomet

a trade name for METHYLTESTOSTERONE.

testosterone

the principal male sex hormone (androgen)
produced in the interstitial cells of the testis and, to
a lesser extent in the ovary. Testosterone is anabolic
and stimulates bone and muscle growth and the
growth of the sexual characteristics. It is also used
as a drug to treat delayed puberty or some cases of
infertility.

tetracaine hydrochloride

a local anaesthetic drug.

tetracosactrin
an analogue of ACTH used as a test of adrenal function. An injection of the drug is given and the resulting rise in serum cortisol is monitored.

tetracyclines
a group of ANTIBIOTIC drugs used to treat a wide range of infections including rickettsial diseases, cholera, brucellosis and most of the sexually transmitted diseases. A trade name is Aureomycin.

tetrahydroaminoacridine
a drug that has been used experimentally to try to improve the situation of people with Alzheimer's disease.

Tetrex
a trade name for TETRACYCLINE.

thalidomide
a drug (Distaval) that was widely advertised as a safe sedative. Thalidomide has since been found useful in the treatment of certain forms of leprosy and Behçet's syndrome.

In 1961 it was found that, when given to pregnant women, it caused severe bodily malformation of the fetus with stunting of the limbs, which were often replaced by short flippers (phocomelia).

Theo-Dur
a trade name for THEOPHYLLINE.

Theograd
a trade name for THEOPHYLLINE.

theophylline
a bronchodilator drug used to treat asthma and to assist in cases of heart failure by increasing the heart rate and reducing oedema by promoting urination. Trade names are Franol and Theograd.

Thephorin
a trade name for the ANTIHISTAMINE drug phenindamine.

Theraderm
a trade name for the anti-acne drug benzoyl peroxide.

thiabendazole
an ANTHELMINTIC drug used to get rid of worms such as Toxocara canis, Strongyloides stercoralis and Trichinella spiralis. A trade name is Mintezol.

thiacetazone
a drug used in conjunction with ISONIAZID in the treatment of tuberculosis.

thiamine
vitamin B_1.

thiazide diuretic drugs
a class of drugs that promote a large outflow of urine and are used for the treatment of fluid retention (oedema). They include chlorothiazide, bendrofluazide and cyclopenthiazide.

thioguanine
a drug used in the treatment of acute myeloblastic leukaemia.

thiomersal
a mercurial antiseptic often used to sterilize eye

471

drops and other solutions. Also known as thimerosal.

thiopentone
a barbiturate drug widely used as a pleasant and rapid induction agent for general anaesthesia. The drug is given by slow intravenous injection. A trade name is Pentothal.

Thioprine
a trade name for AZATHIOPRINE.

thioridazine
an antipsychotic drug used to treat schizophrenia and mania. A trade name is Melleril.

thiouracil
a drug that blocks the synthesis of thyroid hormone and can be used to treat thyroid overactivity.

thioxanthene drug
one of a group of antipsychotic drugs related to the phenothiazines. The group includes flupenthixol and clopenthixol.

thymoxamine
a drug that widens blood vessels (vasodilator) and
may be useful in the management of Raynaud's
disease. A trade name is Opilon.

thyroxine
the principal thyroid hormone. Thyroxine has four
iodine atoms in the molecule and is often known as
T4.

tiaprofenic acid
a non-steroidal anti-inflammatory drug (NSAID) of
the propionic acid group,

ticaricillin
a penicillin-type antibiotic useful for its action
against the organism pseudomonas aeruginosa.

Ticillin
a trade name for TICARCILLIN.

Tiempe
a trade name for TRIMETHOPRIM.

Tigason [W]
a trade name for the retinol antipsoriasis drug etretinate.

Tildiem
a trade name for the calcium channel blocker anti-angina drug diltiazem.

timolol
a beta-blocker drug used to treat high blood pressure and angina pectoris and, in the form of eye drops, to treat glaucoma. A trade name is Betim.

Timoptol
a trade name for eye drops containing the BETA-BLOCKER drug TIMOLOL, used to control glaucoma.

Tinacidin
a trade name for TOLNAFTATE. [O]

Tinaderm-M
a trade name for a mixture of the antifungal drugs

KEY
The symbol [O] indicates that the drug is either available over-the-counter or that an over-the-counter drug with the same active ingredient or ingredients is available.

The symbol [»] indicates the forms in which the drug can be taken.

The symbol [S] sets out side-effects.

The symbol [W] indicates a drug recently withdrawn. These drugs should not be used.

nystatin and tolnaftate, used to treat skin fungus infections.

Tineaderm
a trade name for TOLNAFTATE. [O]

Tineafax
a trade name for TOLNAFTATE. [O]

tinidazole
an antibacterial and antiprotozoal drug similar to
METRONIDAZOLE but with a longer duration of
action.

Tinset
a trade name for the ANTIHISTAMINE drug
oxatomide.

tissue-plasminogen activators
drugs used to dissolve blood clots in the arteries. A
tissue plasminogen activator (TPA) is a naturally
occurring enzyme which can dissolve blood clots.
Since so many serious conditions are caused by
clotting (thrombosis) within the arteries, or by the
breaking free of clots inside veins, clearly a
substance capable of breaking down clots and
allowing a restoration of the blood flow is of major
medical importance.

Other plasminogen activators, such as streptokinase
and urokinase, have been in use for a few years for
this purpose and have achieved some success if
given within an hour or two of the thrombosis. But

TPA appears to have several major advantages over these. It is believed to be the substance responsible for the observed opening up (recanalization) of blood vessels blocked by thrombosis, and its activity is much greater in the presence of mature clot (fibrin) than either streptokinase or urokinase. It can now be produced by genetic engineering techniques and is marketed under the name Activase (altiplase).

Many important studies have now been done on patients with recent coronary thromboses, people with unstable angina and people in whom blood clots have travelled to the lungs causing the dangerous condition of pulmonary embolism. TPA can open up blocked coronary arteries within nineteen to fifty minutes of the injection, restoring the blood supply to the heart muscle and, if the affected area of muscle has not been killed, restoring its function. It can dissolve large clots carried to the lungs from the veins that are responsible for pulmonary embolism and can stop these clots forming (deep vein thrombosis). The drug does not produce antibodies. The results are uniformly excellent and there is no doubt that TPA is an important advance in treatment.

The main side-effect is the tendency to cause bleeding and the drug is dangerous in people who have recently had a stroke, in those with any bleeding tendency and in people with a history of peptic ulcer. The drug does not distinguish between a thrombosis and a naturally occurring sealing plug of clot. So bleeding readily occurs from recent injection sites or at the points of insertion of blood vessel catheters.

Tobralex
a trade name for eye drops containing TOBRAMYCIN.

tobramycin
an ANTIBIOTIC drug similar in use to Gentamicin, but useful in the treatment of gentamicin-resistant infections. A trade name is Nebcin.

tocainide
a drug used to treat a life-threatening tendency to

ventricular fibrillation (cardiac arrest). A trade
name is Tonocard.

tocopherol
one of the forms of vitamin E.

Tofranil
a trade name for IMIPRAMINE.

Tolanase
a trade name for the oral antidiabetic drug
TOLAZAMIDE.

tolazamide
a sulphonylurea drug used to treat maturity-onset,
non-insulin-dependent diabetes.

tolazoline
a drug that causes marked widening (dilatation) of
blood vessels and is used to treat conditions, such
as Raynaud's disease in which blood vessels go into
spasm.

tolbutamide
a drug used in the treatment of maturity-onset, non-insulin-dependent diabetes. A trade name is Rastinon.

Tolectin DS
a trade name for TOLMETIN.

tolmetin
a non-steroidal anti-inflammatory drug (NSAID) used especially for the relief of pain and stiffness in osteoarthritis, rheumatoid arthritis and ankylosing spondylitis. A trade name is Tolectin.

tolnaftate
an antifungal drug used to treat tinea. A trade name is Timoped. [O]

Tonocard
a trade name for the anti-arrhythmic heart drug tocainide.

Topal
a trade name for a mixture of aluminium

hydroxide, alginic acid and magnesium carbonate, used to treat dyspepsia. **[O]**

Topilar
a trade name for the CORTICOSTEROID DRUG fluclorolone, used for local (topical) applications.

Torecan
a trade name for the anti-emetic drug thiethylperazine.

Trancopal
a trade name for the BENZODIAZEPINE anti-anxiety drug chlormezanone.

Trandate
a trade name for the beta-blocker drug LABETALOL.

tranexamic acid
a drug that interferes with the dissolution of blood clot (fibrinolysis) and can be used to prevent bleeding during minor operations such as tooth extraction in people with haemophilia.

481

tranquillizer drugs
drugs used to relieve anxiety or to treat psychotic illness by their muscle-relaxing and anxiety-relieving action. The major ANTIDEPRESSANT and antipsychotic drugs are excluded from this group which includes such drugs as the BENZODIAZEPINES, the BARBITURATES, the BETA-BLOCKER DRUGS and some of the mild HYPNOTIC DRUGS. Other drugs such as Equanil (meprobamate) and Buspar (buspirone) are also used. See also ANTI-ANXIETY DRUGS.

Tranxene
a trade name for the BENZODIAZEPINE anti-anxiety drug clorazepate.

tranylcypromine
a MONOAMINE-OXIDASE INHIBITOR ANTIDEPRESSANT DRUG.

Trasicor
a trade name for the beta-blocker drug oxprenolol.

Tremonil [W]
a trade name for the anticholinergic drug
methixene, used to control symptoms of
Parkinson's disease.

tretinoin
a drug used to treat acne and scaly skin conditions
such as ichthyosis.

triamcinolone
a CORTICOSTEROID DRUG used to treat
inflammatory disorders, asthma, thrombocytopenia
and some forms of leukaemia. A trade name is
Adcortyl.

triamterene
a potassium-sparing diuretic drug used to relieve
the body of excess water and to treat mildly raised
blood pressure. A trade name is Dytide.

triazolam
a BENZODIAZEPINE sedative drug used to relieve
insomnia. A trade name is Halcion.

Trib
a trade name for CO-TRIMOXAZOLE.

Trichozole
a trade name for METRONIDAZOLE.

tricyclic antidepressant drugs
see ANTIDEPRESSANT DRUGS.

Tridesilon
a trade name for the CORTICOSTEROID DRUG desonide, used for local applications.

Tridil
a trade name for GLYCERYL TRINITRATE.

trifluoperazine
an antipsychotic drug used mainly to treat schizophrenia. A trade name is Stelazine.

Trilafon
a trade name for PERPHENAZINE.

Trilisate
a trade name for the anti-inflammatory and pain-killing drug choline magnesium trisalicylate.

Triludan
a trade name for the ANTIHISTAMINE drug terfenadine.

trimeprazine
an ANTIHISTAMINE drug used to relieve itching in allergic conditions and as a sedative for children. A trade name is Vallergan.

trimethoprim
an antibacterial drug commonly used to treat urinary infections. Combined with sulphamethoxazole it is sold as co-trimoxazole (Septrin). A trade name is Bactrim.

trimipramine
a tricyclic ANTIDEPRESSANT DRUG with a strong sedative effect. A trade name is Surmontil.

Trimogal
a trade name for TRIMETHOPRIM.

Triominic
a trade name for a mixture of the nasal
decongestant drug PHENYLPROPANOLAMINE and
the ANTIHISTAMINE drug pheniramine.

Triperidol
a trade name for the antipsychotic drug
trifluperidol.

triple vaccine
a combined vaccine against diphtheria, whooping
cough (pertussis) and tetanus.

Triplopen
a trade name for the penicillin ANTIBIOTIC
benethamine penicillin.

Triprim
a trade name for TRIMETHOPRIM.

triprolidine

an ANTIHISTAMINE drug used to treat allergy and to relieve the symptoms of colds. Trade names are Actidil and Actifed.

Triptafen

a trade name for the tricyclic ANTIDEPRESSANT DRUG amitriptyline and the antipsychotic and anti-emetic drug perphenazine.

tropicamide

a drug used in the form of eye drops to widen (dilate) the pupil so that the inside of the eye can more easily be examined or operated upon. A trade name is Mydriacyl.

Tropium

a trade name for the BENZODIAZEPINE anti-anxiety drug chlordiazepoxide.

Tryptanol

a trade name for AMITRIPTYLINE.

Tryptizol
a trade name for AMITRIPTYLINE.

tryptophan
an ANTIDEPRESSANT DRUG. L-tryptophan, sold in USA as a non-prescription food additive was withdrawn by the American Food and Drugs Administration (FDA) because of reports of a severe muscle disorder apparently caused by an unidentified contaminant. A trade name is Optimax.

Tussinol
a trade name for PHOLCODINE.

Tylex
a trade name for a mixture of the pain-killing drugs CODEINE and PARACETAMOL. [O]

Tyrosets
a trade name for throat lozenges containing the local anaesthetic drug benzocaine.

tyrothricin
an ANTIBIOTIC obtained from the soil bacterium
Bacillus brevis and used by local application to treat
gram positive infections. It is too toxic for internal
use.

Ukidan
a trade name for urokinase, used in the treatment
of thrombosis.

Ulcol
a trade name for SULPHASALAZINE.

Ultralente MC
a trade name for a long-acting INSULIN.

Ultratard
a trade name for a long-acting form of INSULIN.

undecanoic acid
an antifungal drug for local application. A trade
name in Mycil. [O]

> **KEY**
> The symbol [O] indicates that the drug is either available over-the-counter or that an over-the-counter drug with the same active ingredient or ingredients is available.
>
> The symbol [»] indicates the forms in which the drug can be taken.
>
> The symbol [S] sets out side-effects.
>
> The symbol [W] indicates a drug recently withdrawn. These drugs should not be used.

undecylenic acid

an antifungal drug used to treat external fungal infections. A trade name is Tineafax.

Unicap T

a trade name for a multivitamin and mineral preparation.

Unihep

a trade name for the anticoagulant HEPARIN.

Unimycin

a trade name for ANTIBIOTIC drug oxytetracycline.

Uniparin

a trade name for HEPARIN.

Unisomnia

a trade name for NITRAZEPAM.

Univer

a trade name for the CALCIUM CHANNEL BLOCKER, anti-angina drug verapamil.

Urantoin

a trade name for the antibacterial drug nitrofurantoin.

Uremide

a trade name for FRUSEMIDE.

Urex

a trade name for FRUSEMIDE.

Uriben
a trade name for the antibacterial drug nalidixic acid.

Urisal
a trade name for sodium citrate, a drug used to make the urine less acid.

Urispas
a trade name for the urinary ANTISPASMODIC drug flavoxate.

Uromide
a trade name for a mixture of the pain-relieving drug phenazopyridine and the sulphonamide drug sulphaurea, used to treat urinary infections.

ursodeoxycholic acid
a drug used to treat cholesterol gallstones.

[S] *Side-effects are infrequent but include diarrhoea and indigestion. A trade name is Destolit, Ursofalk.*

Ursofalk
a trade name for URSODEOXYCHOLIC ACID.

Uticillin
a trade name for the penicillin-type ANTIBIOTIC
carfecillin.

Utovian
a trade name for NORETHISTERONE.

Vaginyl
a trade name for the drug METRONIDAZOLE.

Valcote
a trade name for SODIUM VALPROATE.

Valium
a trade name for DIAZEPAM.

Vallergan
a trade name for the ANTIHISTAMINE drug
TRIMEPRAZINE.

Valoid
a trade name for the ANTI-EMETIC ANTIHISTAMINE drug cyclizine.

Vancocin
a trade name for the ANTIBIOTIC VANCOMYCIN.

vancomycin
an ANTIBIOTIC drug which is effective against many gram positive bacteria. It is toxic and its use is limited to infections that fail to respond to the more common ANTIBIOTICS.

Varidase
a trade name for a mixture of STREPTOKINASE and streptodornase used locally to remove blood clots and organic debris from wounds.

Vascardin
a trade name for the nitrate VASODILATOR drug, isosorbide dinitrate, used to treat angina pectoris.

vasoconstrictor drugs
drugs which cause the smooth muscle in the walls

of arteries to contract so that the vessel is narrowed and the rate of blood flow though it reduced. The natural hormones adrenaline and noradrenaline act on particular alpha-adrenergic receptors to cause vasoconstriction. Both nicotine and cocaine are powerful vasoconstrictors and the former has been implicated in the gangrene-producing disease thromboangiitis obliterans (Buerger's disease). See also DECONGESTANT DRUGS, SYMPATHOMIMETIC DRUGS.

vasodilator drugs

drugs which cause arteries to widen, improving the blood flow through them. Vasodilator drugs are often valuable, but sometimes cause alarming effects by lowering the blood pressure too much. They include NITRATE AND NITRITE DRUGS, drugs such as prazosin and hydralazine, and CALCIUM CHANNEL BLOCKERS such as nifepidine.

Veganin

a trade name for a mixture of the pain-killing drugs ASPIRIN, CODEINE and PARACETAMOL. [O]

Velbe
a trade name for the anticancer drug VINBLASTINE.

Velosulin
a trade name for INSULIN.

venene
a mixture of snake venoms used to produce a
general antidote (antivenin).

Ventide
a trade name for a mixture of the steroid drug
beclomethasone and the BRONCHODILATOR drug
salbutamol, used to control asthma.

Ventolin
a trade name for the bronchodilator drug
SALBUTAMOL.

Veractil
a trade name for the antipsychotic drug
methotrimeprazine.

Veradil
a trade name for VERAPAMIL.

verapamil
a calcium channel blocker drug used to correct
irregularities in the heart beat.

Vermox
a trade name for the anthelmintic drug
MEBENDAZOLE.

Vertigon
a trade name for the phenothiazine anti-emetic
drug prochlorperazine.

Vibramycin
a trade name for the tetracycline ANTIBIOTIC
doxycycline.

vidarabine
a drug that inhibits DNA synthesis and is used to
treat Herpes simplex, shingles and cytomegalovirus
infections. A trade name is Vira-A.

vinblastine
an anticancer drug used mainly in the treatment of Hodgkin's disease and other lymphomas.

vinca alkaloids
drugs that bind to the protein tubulin that forms the fine strands in cells that pull the chromosomes apart in cell division (mitosis). The effect is to interfere with mitosis and is thus of value in the treatment of various cancers. Vinca alkaloids are used especially in acute leukaemias and malignant lymphomas. The include vinblastine and vincristine.

Vincent's powders
a trade name for ASPIRIN. [O]

vincristine, vindesine
vinca alkaloid anticancer drugs used to treat leukaemia.

Viokase
a trade name for PANCREATIN.

viomycin

an ANTIBIOTIC drug used in cases of tuberculosis that resist standard treatment.

Vira-A

a trade name for VIDARABINE.

Virormone

a trade name for the male sex hormone drug testosterone.

Visclair

a trade name for the mucus-dissolving drug methylcysteine.

Visken

a trade name for the beta-blocker drug pindolol.

Visopt

a trade name for eye drops containing PHENYLEPHRINE and HYPROMELLOSE.

Voltaren, Voltarol

trade names for DICLOFENAC.

warfarin
an ANTICOAGULANT drug used to treat abnormal
or undesired clotting of the blood.

Welldorm
a trade name for the sleeping drug
dichloralphenazone.

Wellferon
a trade name for an INTERFERON preparation.
Interferons are proteins used in the treatment of
cancer.

Winsprin
a trade name for ASPIRIN. [O]

xamoterol
a beta-adrenergic agonist drug which is used in the
treatment of long-term mild heart failure. A trade
name is Corwin.

Xylocaine, Xylocard
trade names for the local anaesthetic drug
lignocaine.

xylometazoline
a decongestant drug to relieve blocked nose.

yohimbine
an alkaloid adrenoreceptor antagonist derived
from the yohimbe tree. It lowers blood pressure
and controls arousal and anxiety and has been used
to treat both physical and psychogenic impotence.

Yomesan
a trade name for the ANTHELMINTIC drug
niclosamide.

Yutopar
a trade name for the womb-relaxing drug
RITODRINE.

Zaditen
a trade name for the anti-allergic drug ketotifen.

Zadstat
a trade name for METRONIDAZOLE.

zalcitabine

a drug, similar to didanosine, that can block the action of the enzyme reverse transcriptase in the human immunodeficiency virus (HIV), the cause of AIDS. This action interferes with the replication of the virus in the human T-cell. Zalcitabine cannot cure AIDS but is used in an attempt to prolong life.

Zantac

a trade name for the stomach acid reducing drug RANITIDINE.

Zarontin

a trade name for the ANTI-EPILEPSY drug ethosuximide.

zidovudine

an antiviral drug used to try to retard the progress of AIDS. Also known as azidothymidine or AZT. A trade name is Retrovir.

zimelidine

an ANTIDEPRESSANT DRUG.

Zinamide

a trade name for the antituberculosis drug pyrazinamide.

Zincaps

a trade name for a ZINC preparation.

Zincfrin

a trade name for eye drops containing the ASTRINGENT zinc sulphate and PHENYLEPHRINE.

zinc oxide

a white powder with mild ASTRINGENT properties used as a dusting powder or incorporated into creams or ointments and used as a bland skin application. Mixed with oil of cloves, zinc oxide forms an effective and pain-relieving temporary dressing for a tooth cavity. **[O]**

Zinnat

a trade name for the cephalosporin ANTIBIOTIC cefuroxime.

Zonulysin
a trade name for the protein-splitting enzyme
alpha-chymotrypsin, made up in a solution to
dissole the suspensory ligament of the crystalline
lens, prior to the removal of a cataract of the eye.

Zovirax
a trade name for the antiviral drug ACYCLOVIR. [O]

Zyloprim
a trade name for ALLOPURINOL that blocks the
formation of uric acid and is used in the prevention
of gout.

Zyloric
a trade name for the drug ALLOPURINOL.

First aid

What to do in a medical emergency

CONTENTS

First aid 508

LIFE-THREATENING SITUATIONS

The air supply 511

Mouth-to-mouth artificial respiration 516

Unconsciousness and the recovery position 520

Heart stopped 522

EMERGENCY: Cardiac arrest 524

Choking 530

EMERGENCY: Choking 534

Bleeding 535

EMERGENCY: Bleeding 537

Shock 538

EMERGENCY: Preventing shock 539

Near drowning 540

EMERGENCY: Near drowning 541

Poisoning   542

EMERGENCY: Poisoning   543

Burns   552

EMERGENCY: Burns   553

Heat disorders   555

EMERGENCY: Heat stroke   558

Electric shock   560

EMERGENCY: Electric shock   561

NON-LIFE-THREATENING SITUATIONS

Corrosives in the eye   562

Foreign body in the eye   564

Fractures   567

Nose bleeds   570

Fainting   573

FIRST AID

The immediate assistance given to an injured person by someone who happens to be present is often more important than expert medical care given later. In some cases it is only the person on the spot who can save a life or prevent serious long-term disability.

There is, of course, no legal responsibility on anyone to do anything, but common humanity demands that every responsible person should be ready to help.

Whether this help is useful or not depends on whether the helper knows what to do. The possession of a few basic facts and a little vital knowledge about procedure can make the difference between saving a life and standing around watching a fellow human die.

So it is necessary to learn about the priorities and how to act accordingly. There are only a few really essential points and these should be known by everyone. Apart from these, most of the detail contained in first aid manuals is unim-

Never:

- delay getting seriously injured people to hospital or waste time on their trivial injuries or fancy bandages;

- heap an injured person with blankets and clothes, simply because they are shivering. This can precipitate a state of deadly surgical shock;

- apply a tourniquet to control minor bleeding. Healthy limbs can become gangrenous and are lost;

- fail to appreciate the critical importance of ensuring that the injured person can breathe properly. Often the airway is ignored while pressure points are searched for to control relatively unimportant bleeding from small arteries.

portant and may even direct attention away from what really matters. Most accidents occur in the home and far more deaths and serious disability occur from home accidents than from car or other accidents away from home. So it is up to all of us to know what to do.

In all cases, get medical help as soon as possible, but if action is urgently needed to ensure breathing, this has priority. If necessary, send someone else to phone for an ambulance. Never delay arranging to call an ambulance, however.

Ambulance paramedics are highly trained and experienced in all measures necessary to save life in emergency, and they carry all the necessary equipment. They can pass tracheal tubes to maintain an airway; can carry out cardiac compression and defibrillation in cases of cardiac arrest; can start a transfusion when required; and they have the equipment and skills to control serious bleeding.

LIFE-THREATENING SITUATIONS

The air supply

Successful first aid in critical situations depends on understanding and applying priorities. The first and most urgent requirement is for air, so that the brain can get its oxygen supply. It usually takes a long time to bleed to death, but total deprivation of air for even a few minutes is fatal or can cause brain damage. A person who cannot

---

The Priorities

Remember ABC

AIRWAY,

BREATHING *and*

CIRCULATION

---

breathe for whatever reason, or whose airway is obstructed, is dying, and everything else is secondary to the critical requirement of restoring the supply of air. Brain damage from partial deprivation of air is usually more serious than any other kind of injury.

Obstruction to the airway can occur in many ways. In an unconscious person the tongue may fall back and block the air passage. Blood, vomited food, even collected saliva can block the airway. The casualty may have choked on a large piece of food accidentally inhaled into the voice box in the neck (see Choking, page 530). Whatever the cause, the situation is critical and the obstruction must be relieved at once.

Clear the mouth with your finger. Remove loose dentures and all foreign material. Mop out the mouth with a handkerchief. Bend the head as far back as possible and push the lower jaw upwards until the teeth are clenched. Check for breathing. If occurring, and the casualty is unconscious, maintain the position of the head. If there is no breathing, start mouth-to-mouth respiration (see page 516).

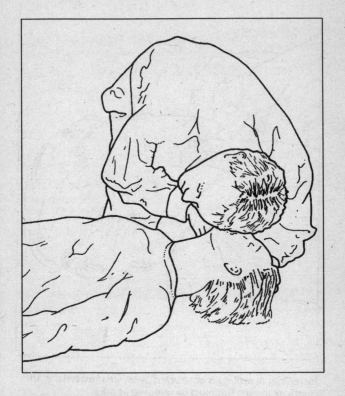

The first priority is to ensure that the unconscious person is breathing. **513**

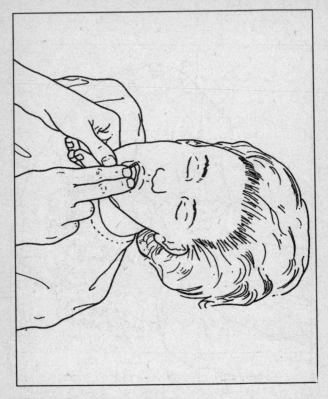

Sometimes breathing is obstructed by vomited material in the mouth or throat. This must be removed at once.

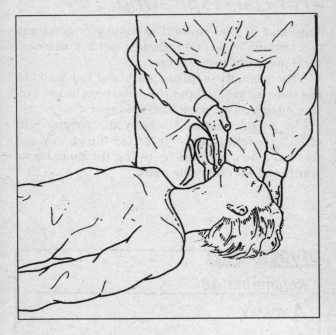

This position will allow free and safe breathing in most unconscious subjects by pulling the relaxed tongue forward off the back of the throat. It is still vital to check that the airway is clear. Do not tilt the head back if there is any possibility that the neck is broken.

Mouth-to-mouth artificial respiration

The 'kiss of life' (mouth-to-mouth respiration) can be done by a single rescuer, but is much easier if there are two or more.

The casualty is turned on his or her back on the floor or ground and the clearness of the airway ensured (see page 512).

In an unconscious person the tongue will often have fallen back to obstruct the airway and this must be overcome by tilting the head backwards and elevating the chin.

The Priorities

Remember ABC

AIRWAY,

BREATHING and

CIRCULATION

> ### Remember
> **If there is any possibility of a broken neck, the head should never be moved.**

With the head kept in the extended position by one hand under the chin, the other hand is used to pinch the nose. The rescuer now applies his or her wide open lips to the mouth of the victim, making a good seal around the casualty's mouth.

Regular full breaths are now blown in hard, at first as quickly as possible, then at a rate of sixteen to twenty blows a minute. If done properly, the casualty's chest will rise well with each blow, and between blows the air will come out.

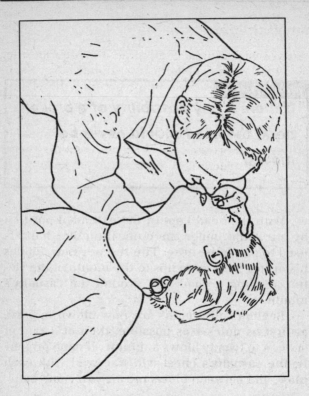

The head must be maintained in the extended position. The subject's nose must be pinched before blowing into the open mouth. Check that the chest rises and listen for the air coming out again.

Small children

When respirating a small child it is often best to put the mouth over both mouth and nose. Keep this up for at least an hour, or until the victim breathes spontaneously.

It is important to ensure that air is actually going in and out and that the chest is rising and falling. If there are no chest movements there may be obstruction in the larynx (see section on choking, page 530).

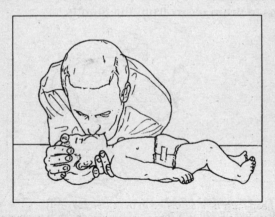

When giving artificial respiration to babies and small children it is often best to blow into both nose and mouth simultaneously.

Unconsciousness and the recovery position

An unconscious, but breathing casualty may vomit and obstruct their airway. The tongue may fall back and do the same. To prevent obstruction, such a person should be placed in the recovery position while you wait for help to arrive. The recovery position keeps the victim still, makes the jaw and tongue fall forward so that breathing is free, and allows vomit or secretions to drain easily from the mouth.

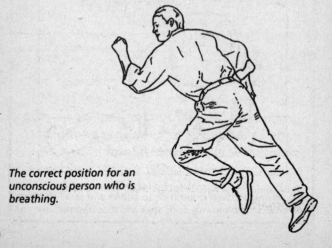

The correct position for an unconscious person who is breathing.

The recovery position

Here is what to do

- The unconscious person should be turned on their front, head turned to one side, and one leg bent to prevent rolling.
- Check at frequent intervals that breathing is continuing.
- If breathing stops, turn the casualty over and start mouth-to-mouth respiration (see page 516).

Warning

If the injury was such that a fracture of the spine is probable, there is danger that in turning the casualty further damage may be done to the spinal cord, causing permanent paralysis or even death. In such a case, any movement, except under the supervision of a skilled and knowledgeable person, is dangerous.

Heart stopped (cardiac arrest)

Oxygen to the brain is the literally vital requirement and this implies that the blood, which carries the oxygen, is circulating. If the heart has stopped beating (cardiac arrest), the blood has stopped circulating, so the heart must be started again, or must be squeezed repeatedly so that the blood is circulated.

A heart attack may stop the heart. Often the heart is not severely damaged – the arteries supplying the heart (the coronary arteries) may simply have gone into spasm – but if nothing is done the person will die. A knowledge of cardio-pulmonary resuscitation will save a life in such a case and may restore a person to normal. Out of hospital, there is never time to summon medical assistance.

Cardiac arrest does not necessarily mean that the heart has stopped contracting completely. In cardiac arrest, the lower pumping chambers (the ventricles) are no longer maintaining the circulation of the blood around the body.

The heart may be stopped or it may be in a state of rapid, ineffectual twitching, called ventricular fibrillation. In either case, no pumping action is occurring and, unless something is done within two or three minutes, death is inevitable from failure of the oxygen and sugar supply to the brain.

Within seconds of a cardiac arrest, consciousness is lost, the breathing becomes rapid and shallow and soon stops. No pulse can be felt and no heart sounds heard. Within minutes, the pupils of the eyes become very wide (dilated), and the skin turns bluish (cyanosis).

To save the person's life, immediate artificial respiration and cardiac massage are needed (cardio-pulmonary resuscitation).

The Priorities

Remember ABC

AIRWAY,

BREATHING *and*

CIRCULATION

EMERGENCY

CARDIAC ARREST: 1

Here is what to do

- If there is someone else around, send them to call an ambulance or get medical help.
- Check if the subject is conscious. If so, the heart has not stopped.
- Check for breathing. Put your ear close to the subject's mouth and watch the chest for breathing movement. If you hear or feel the breath or see the chest moving, the heart has not stopped.
- Clear the mouth and throat with your finger. Make sure there is no obstruction and that the tongue is well forward.
- Position the patient flat on their back on the floor.
- Tilt the head back by pushing the chin upwards and lift the jaw forward.
- If there is no breathing, pinch the subject's nostrils closed with the fingers, seal your mouth tightly around their mouth, and blow until the subject's chest rises well.

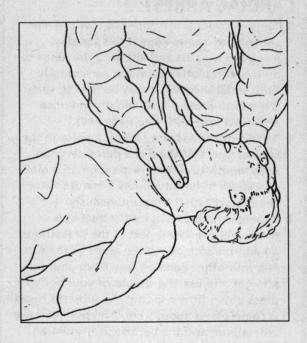

To feel a pulse in the neck, press firmly backwards with the fingertips between the Adam's apple and the front border of the prominent angled muscle.

CARDIAC ARREST: 2

- Remove your mouth and listen for the air coming out again. Repeat this steadily, using full breaths and allowing the lungs to deflate completely between each breath. With small children, it may be best to seal the mouth around both mouth and nose and blow into both (see page 519).

- Do this five times and feel for a pulse in the subject's neck. If there is a pulse, carry on with mouth-to-mouth respiration, at a rate of sixteen to twenty blows a minute, until the subject breathes spontaneously.

- If there is no pulse, place the heel of one hand over the lower part of the breastbone a hand-breadth above the angle of the ribs. Put your other hand on top. Keep your arms straight and use the weight of your body to press down firmly so that the subject's heart is compressed about 5 cm (2 in) between the breastbone and the backbone. In children much less force is needed. Do this, evenly and smoothly, fifteen times in ten seconds, and then give two full mouth-to-mouth ventilations.

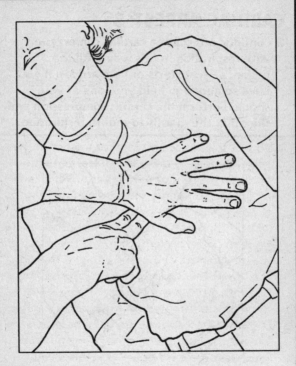

Heart compression is done over the lower half of the breastbone, centrally. Place the centre of the hand two finger-breadths above the angle of the ribs.

CARDIAC ARREST: 3

● Continue alternating cardiac compression with respiration in this way until the patient's heart starts or help arrives. If you have someone to help you, one of you should perform the cardiac compression and the other the mouth-to-mouth respiration.

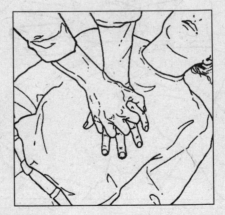

Keep the arms straight so that the weight of the body is used to depress the breastbone about two inches. Do this fifteen times in ten seconds then give two full mouth-to-mouth blows. Continue until help arrives or the subject recovers.

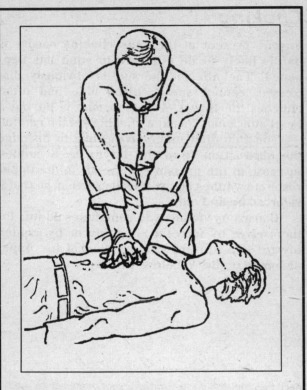

This shows the correct attitude for heart compression.
Note that the arms must be kept straight.

Choking

Anyone present at the time choking occurs is hardly likely to be unaware of what has happened. The affected person is obviously distressed, cannot speak, turns blue and often clutches the throat. A person who is having a heart attack can speak; a choking person cannot.

The Heimlich manoeuvre aims to dislodge the obstruction from the larynx by a sudden increase in the pressure of the air in the upper respiratory tubes below the obstruction, so that it is forced up and out.

Conscious victims can sometimes do this for themselves by forceful coughing or by sudden inward and upward compression of the upper abdomen in the 'V' below the ribs.

Remember

The recommended first aid in choking is the abdominal thrust (see pages 532-533). This is also called the Heimlich manoeuvre. Slapping the back is of little value. Remember that a person in this situation is dying. Mere details like bruised or torn muscles are of no concern by comparison with the over-riding necessity to restore the airway.

The Priorities

Remember ABC

AIRWAY,

BREATHING *and*

CIRCULATION

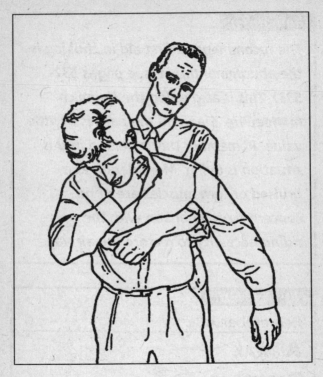

By suddenly compressing the air in the chest in the Heimlich manoeuvre it is often possible to blow out a foreign body causing obstruction.

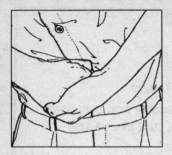

The thrust should be inwards and upwards and must be vigorous

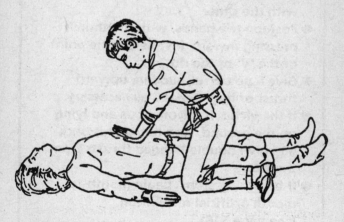

The same effect as the Heimlich can be achieved by an inwards and upwards double-handed thrust.

EMERGENCY

Choking

Here is what to do

- Get behind the casualty and put your arms around them, just above the waist.
- Make a fist with one hand and grasp it with the other.
- Position the hands, with the thumb pressing inward, just below the point of the 'V' of the ribs.
- Give a powerful, sudden, upward thrust or hug. Repeat, as necessary.
- If the victim is unconscious and lying on the ground, turn him on his back and give double-handed thrusts from the front.
- If breathing stops, begin mouth-to-mouth artificial respiration (see page 516).

Bleeding

After ensuring air supply and circulation, the next priority is the control of severe bleeding. This, too, is largely in the interests of a continued supply of oxygen to the brain. If there is not enough blood, insufficient oxygen will be carried to the brain. External bleeding is easily controlled, as will be seen. Internal bleeding requires surgical intervention, so get the injured person to hospital as quickly as possible.

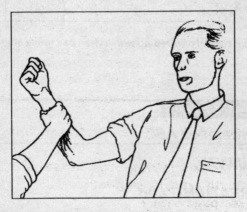

The correct method of controlling bleeding is to apply immediate, direct, firm pressure to the bleeding area. Apply pressure first, then look for a pad. Elevating the part can help.

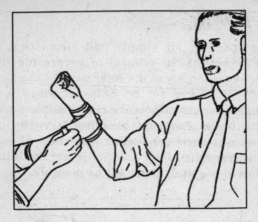

Maintain control of bleeding with a clean pad firmly bound in place.

The Priorities

Remember ABC

AIRWAY,

BREATHING and

CIRCULATION

! *EMERGENCY*

Bleeding

Here is what to do

- The first aid management of obvious external bleeding is easy. Apply direct pressure to the bleeding area and maintain it.
- Use your hand until you have time to think.
- Look for something with which to make a pad.
- Apply it firmly and fix it in place, using an encircling tie.
- Try to elevate the bleeding part and to keep it at rest, so that a clot can form.
- Make sure you can see what is happening and that continued bleeding is not just seeping into the clothes.
- Direct pressure, properly maintained, will stop almost any bleeding.
- Forget about pressure points and never use tourniquets. These can lead to gangrene.

Shock

Severe injury often leads to a dangerous condition in which the blood, instead of circulating normally through tight arteries and veins, forms useless pools or depots in widely dilated vessels in the skin, digestive system and legs.

This is called surgical shock and it has nothing to do with fright. Shock is another way in which the brain can be deprived of oxygen, and the prevention of shock is the third priority.

Prevention of shock is simple. It is essential for the victim to make the fullest use of the blood available and this must not be wasted by flushing the skin or filling the legs.

! EMERGENCY

Preventing shock

- Do not pile up the injured person with blankets. Shivering and complaints of cold do not matter. Use one blanket only.
- Elevate the legs, if possible, to improve the blood return to the heart and brain.
- A person in surgical shock desperately needs more fluid and a drip, even of saline solution can be life-saving. Ambulance paramedics can give this.
- Do not give anything by mouth, unless the injury is limited to minor burns.

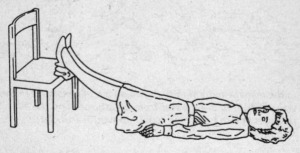

By raising the legs, vital blood can be made available to the heart and brain.

Near-drowning

Near-drowning is another important cause of oxygen deprivation and, again, urgency is of the essence.

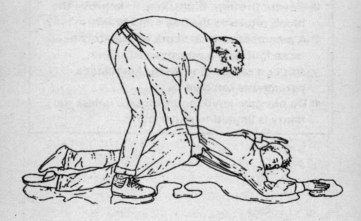

In the management of near-drowning a preliminary lift in this way will help to drain water from the stomach and the air passages before beginning mouth-to-mouth artificial respiration.

EMERGENCY

Near-drowning

Here is what to do

- Mouth-to-mouth artificial respiration must be started at once (see page 516), even before the victim is out of the water, if this is possible.
- If the abdomen is distended with water, the victim should be placed face down and then lifted with the hands under the midriff.
- Clear the airway, check for breathing and pulse. If no pulse is felt, begin cardiopulmonary resuscitation (see Heart stopped, pages 522-529).
- Survival is possible after long periods of immersion in cold water because the lowered temperature reduces the body's requirements for oxygen and brain fuel.

541

Poisoning

There is no first aid for poisoning, unless the victim is unconscious. In this case put him or her in the recovery position (see page 520) and get to hospital, together with all available evidence of the type of poisoning – empty bottles, syringes, samples of vomit, tablets, plants or berries – as soon as possible.

About poisons

Poisons are substances which can injure or kill living organisms when taken in small dosage. The matter of dosage is important because the great majority of substances, even some of those taken as nutrients, are poisons if taken in sufficient amount.

We commonly take very small quantities of very poisonous substances and suffer little or no ill-effects. It is a mistake to believe that most, or even many, poisons accumulate in the body until dangerous levels are reached.

The level in the body is almost always determined by the average intake and reaches a stable state depending on the intake. Usually this level is much too low to do any harm.

! EMERGENCY

Poisoning

Here is what to do

● Do not make the victim vomit.

● Do not give anything by mouth.

● Just get him or her to hospital by any means, with the minimum delay.

● Inform the ambulance people that it is a poisoning case and state whether or not the victim is conscious.

● If going by car, get someone to telephone the hospital casualty department and warn them.

Almost all drugs are poisonous if taken in excess, but are safe if taken in correct dosage under medical supervision. Adult doses may be

543

poisonous to children. Some drugs are especially dangerous in excess and have to be used with special care. Drugs used in the treatment of cancer are capable of destroying living cells, but can be used because their effect on cancer cells is greater than on healthy cells. Nevertheless, they are very toxic.

It is impossible to list all the poisonous substances with which one might come in contact. Some substances, however, are commonly accessible and are particularly toxic and dangerous. Here are some of these, arranged under categories.

Poisons in the home

◆ ammonia
◆ liquid bleach
◆ toilet-bowl cleaning powder or liquid
◆ fungus-killing liquids
◆ oven-cleaning liquids and sprays
◆ corrosive agents, such as acids, alkalis, bleaches and disinfectants
◆ rust removers
◆ paint strippers

- spot removers, especially if inhaled
- sterilizing fluids such as phenols or cresol
- various liquid glues, if inhaled
- coumarin and warfarin rat and mouse poisons
- methylated spirits
- rubbing alcohol
- antifreeze
- drugs

Poisons in the garden and countryside

- organophosphate weedkillers, such as paraquat
- Insecticides, such as Parathion and Malathion
- laburnum berries
- yew
- deadly nightshade
- common inkcap mushroom
- deathcap mushroom
- 'magic' mushrooms
- deadly agaric mushroom

Drug overdose

This occurs most commonly as a suicide attempt or by people seeking to modify their state of mind. Most drug overdoses occur as a result of 'recreational' use.

Occasionally, drug overdose occurs by accident. The most common drugs to be taken in overdose, with brief notes on their effects, include:

heroin and morphine
vomiting, depressed breathing, pin-point pupils

cocaine (Crack)
excitement, euphoria, restlessness, feelings of power, tremor, wide pupils, fast pulse, overbreathing, cardiac arrest

amphetamines (Benzedrine, Dexedrine)
jumpiness, excitement, confusion, aggression, hallucinations

barbiturates (Amytal, Luminal, Seconal)
drowsiness, coma, hypothermia, slow and shallow breathing

> ### The Priorities
>
> *Remember ABC*
>
> **A**IRWAY,
>
> **B**REATHING and
>
> **C**IRCULATION

benzodiazepines (Valium, Librium)
staggering, dizziness, drowsiness, shallow
breathing

beta blockers (Sectral, Visken, Angilol)
digoxin (Lanoxin)
very slow pulse, collapse, drowsiness, delirium,
seizures, cardiac arrest, nausea, vomiting,
diarrhoea, yellow vision, slow irregular pulse

iron (Ferrocap, Ferromyn)
abdominal pain, nausea, vomiting, rapid pulse,
black stools

lithium (Camcolit, Priadel)
nausea, vomiting, apathy, tremor, muscle twitching,
convulsions

NSAIDs (Brufen, Ebufac)
nausea, vomiting, abdominal pain, headache, rapid
breathing, disorientation, jerking eyes, seizures,
drowsiness, coma, cardiac arrest

paracetamol (Panadol)
nausea and vomiting. After thirty-six hours, acute
liver failure which is often fatal

salicylates (Aspirin)
deafness, ringing in the ears, blurring of vision,
profuse sweating, cardiac arrest. Coma in children

tricyclic antidepressants (Tofranil, Tryptizol)
dry mouth, wide pupils, inability to urinate,
hallucinations, twitching, loss of consciousness

Poisonous animals

A few animals, insects and marine creatures produce toxins harmful to man in the doses normally acquired. These include:

- ◆ venomous snakes
- ◆ sea snakes
- ◆ ciguatera (an alga eaten by fish in the Pacific and Caribbean)
- ◆ certain shellfish contaminated by toxic protozoa
- ◆ puffer fish
- ◆ sting rays
- ◆ scorpion fish
- ◆ cone shell molluscs
- ◆ jelly-fish
- ◆ land scorpions
- ◆ centipedes
- ◆ a few tropical spiders

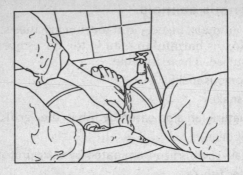

Animal bites and abrasions should be washed thoroughly under running water to remove as much bacterial contamination as possible.

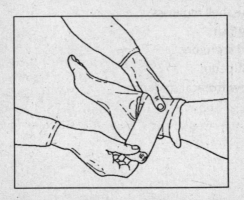

Such wounds should then be covered with a clean dressing.

Industrial poisons

Many inorganic compounds are poisonous, notably:

- the salts of the heavy metals, such as lead, iron, arsenic, gold, silver and mercury;
- strong acids and alkalis, mainly by exerting severe corrosive effects on tissues;
- hundreds of synthetic organic substances;
- many solvents;
- most of the highly reactive gases such as chlorine, bromine, ammonia, hydrogen sulphide and hydrocyanic acid.

Industrial first aid centres are familiar with the relevant toxic substances and with their particular dangers. In some cases antidotes are available. Poison centres exist in most large towns, from which advice can be obtained by telephone. Consult the local telephone directory or directory enquiries.

Burns

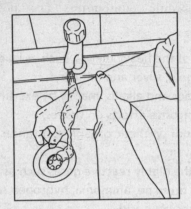

Burn cooling. Tissue damage is caused by heat. Immediate and prolonged cooling under a cold tap can greatly reduce the degree of injury.

Remember

Heat destroys tissue and immediate cooling is the only measure that can help. So get the part under the cold tap and keep it there.

552

EMERGENCY

Burns

Here is what to do

● Get the fire out and cool the burned area as quickly as possible.

● Chemical burns need prolonged washing. You cannot overdo this.

● Do not burst blisters.

● Do not apply any medication, grease, oil or anything else to a severe burn.

● Burns rapidly lead to loss of fluid from the blood and this has to be replaced.

A moderately burned conscious person is the only kind of casualty who should be given plenty of fluids by mouth.

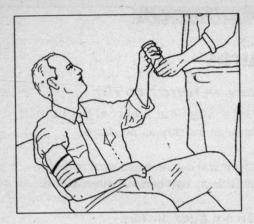

A conscious person with extensive burns should be given plenty of fluids by mouth.

The Priorities

Remember ABC

AIRWAY,

BREATHING and

CIRCULATION

Heat disorders

The body produces considerable heat when fuel (glucose and fatty acids) is slowly burned (oxidized) to provide biochemical energy. During strenuous exercise, there is a large increase in heat production from this source and from muscle action. Heat is also gained from the environment when the external temperature exceeds that of the body.

If the external temperature is low, the body conserves heat by shutting down the blood vessels in the skin, and if additional heat is needed, the muscles shiver. If the body temperature rises too high, the skin vessels open up, causing the skin to flush so that heat is lost. In addition, the evaporation of sweat from the surface of the skin has a highly efficient cooling effect by drawing the latent heat of evaporation from the body.

These mechanisms are controlled by heat-regulating centres in the part of the base of the brain called the hypothalamus, which lies just above the pituitary gland. The temperature-regulating centres monitor the blood heat and respond at once to changes. In fever from disease, abnormal substances in the blood reset the thermostat in the hypothalamus at a higher level and the body responds by regarding normal temperature as too low and turning on more heat production. Various disorders of heat regulation can occur.

Heat cramps

These are due to abnormal loss of sodium from excessive sweating and inadequate replacement. They usually occur after strenuous exercise in conditions of high ambient temperature. The onset is often sudden and incapacitating with hard spasm of the leg, arm or abdominal muscles. Heat cramps are usually rapidly relieved by drinking plenty of fluid containing a little salt. Prevention is easy, if the danger is understood and a good fluid and salt intake ensured.

Remember

The treatment of heat exhaustion is urgent replacement of fluid, by mouth, if possible, or by intravenous infusion if the subject is in coma.

Heat exhaustion

This is simply due to excessive loss of water from the body, so that there is insufficient fluid to maintain the circulation. It is a form of shock and the signs are similar to those of severe blood loss. There is:

◆ weakness;
◆ fatigue;
◆ collapse;
◆ pale clammy skin;
◆ a slow, very weak pulse;
◆ abnormally low blood pressure;
◆ sometimes unconsciousness.

The temperature is usually below normal.

Heat exhaustion occurs when fluid loss from sweating substantially exceeds the intake. The idea that one can be trained to manage on low water intake is as dangerous as it is naïve, and there has been a regular annual death rate, in military circles, from the efforts of Officers and NCOs acting on this mistaken belief.

EMERGENCY

Heat stroke

Heat stroke is a medical emergency. The rising temperature causes brain damage which worsens with duration and level and, if the victim survives, this damage is often irreversible. A rectal temperature of 41° C (106° F) is a sign of grave danger.

● The treatment is to get the temperature down by any available means.

● The whole body should be immersed in cold water and ice-packs and fans used to supplement the cooling.

● The temperature must be monitored continuously and not allowed to drop below 38°C (101°F) as excess cooling may convert hyperthermia to hypothermia.

Heat stroke

Heat hyperpyrexia, or heat stroke, is the most dangerous of all the heat disorders. It occurs when the temperature-regulating centres are unable to cope with excessive heat production, as may occur from excessive exertion in very hot conditions, or when, as a result of disease or other causes, they fail altogether to control the temperature of the body.

The temperature rises rapidly and the situation quickly becomes critical. Initially, there may be warning indications in the form of faintness, dizziness, headache, dry skin, absence of sweating, thirst and nausea. Later there may be lethargy and confusion or agitation progressing to epileptic-like fits, coma and death.

The Priorities

Remember ABC

AIRWAY,

BREATHING and

CIRCULATION

Electric shock

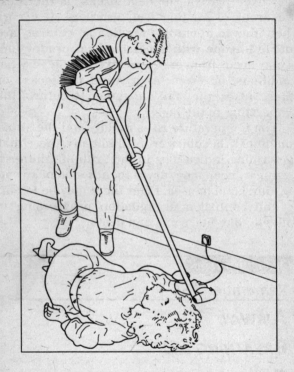

Use an insulating object such as a broom handle to separate the electrical equipment from the shocked person, or pull out the plug, before touching the victim.

EMERGENCY

Electric shock

Here is what to do

- Electric injuries are made worse by continuing flow of current. Switch off, if possible.

- Do not touch the victim until current is off or contact broken.

- Move victim from current source with a broom-handle, a wooden chair, a dry cloth or a plastic garment.

- If the victim is unconscious, has stopped breathing and has no pulse, start cardiac arrest procedure.

- If the victim is breathing and has a pulse place in the recovery position (see page 520).

NON-LIFE-THREATENING SITUATIONS

Corrosives in the eyes

Although there is no danger to life, this does call for urgent action if damage to vision is to be

> ### Remember
>
> *Ideally, a water-tap should be run on to the open eye or eyes, or a hand-shower directed on to them, for ten minutes or longer. The longer the interval between the accident and the start of the wash, the longer it should be continued. If water is not available, any bland fluid, including urine, should be used.*

avoided. The accidental contamination of the eyes with corrosive chemicals such as lime or other alkalis, or strong acids calls for immediate, vigorous, and prolonged washing with a large quantity of water, so that the chemical can be diluted and washed off before it has time to cause permanent damage to the transparency of the corneas.

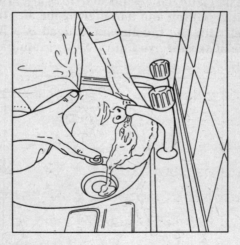

Corrosive substances in the eye can be very damaging. Eyesight can be saved if these are properly washed out without delay. Prolonged washing directly under a tap is one of the best methods. If necessary, the eye should be held open.

Foreign body in eye

This is a fairly common hazard, especially in industrial environments. The danger depends largely on the velocity with which the foreign body strikes the eye. A penetrating foreign body must always be suspected if the activity at the time might have produced high-speed fragments.

Especially dangerous activities are grinding, turning, milling and hammering metal. The cold chisel with the mushroomed head is a prolific cause of serious eye injury. X-ray examination is

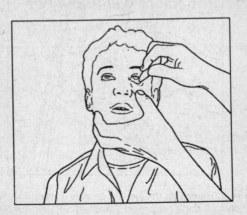

Foreign bodies in the eye can often be safely removed on the point of a folded tissue or clean handkerchief.

Remember

Attempts to remove corneal foreign bodies may cause further damage and if the foreign body is central, permanent visual loss may result. A wash with an eyebath may occasionally be successful, but specialist advice will usually be necessary.

mandatory in all such cases for a retained metallic intra-ocular foreign body will usually do serious harm to the eye – often after many months.

Most foreign bodies do not penetrate the eye, but lodge on the membrane covering the white of the eye (the conjunctiva) or behind the lids. Foreign bodies on the transparent front lens (the cornea) cause exquisite pain and intense awareness and induce an uncontrollable tendency to squeeze the lids – an activity calculated to increase the pain. Unless sharp and on the cen-

tre of the cornea, however, superficial foreign
bodies are unlikely to do much harm.

◆ A foreign body behind the upper lid may
  sometimes be dislodged by grasping the lashes
  and pulling it down over the lower lid so that the
  lower lashes can brush it off.
◆ Eversion of the upper lid, to examine its
  underside, may be very easy or very difficult
  depending on whether or not the affected
  person trusts the operator. A cotton bud, or even
  a matchstick, will help.
◆ Get the victim to look down, pull the upper lid
  lashes downward, press the tip of the bud
  against the skin, one centimetre above the lid
  margin, and pull on the lashes, outwards and
  then upwards. This can be done quite gently and
  painlessly so long as the victim keeps still and
  continues to look down.
◆ Superficial foreign bodies may safely be removed
  from the conjunctiva using a piece of paper tissue
  folded to a point.

Fractures

Broken bones call for immobilization. Unnecessary movement may cause increased loss of blood and may precipitate surgical shock. Effective emergency splints always need to be longer than might be expected.

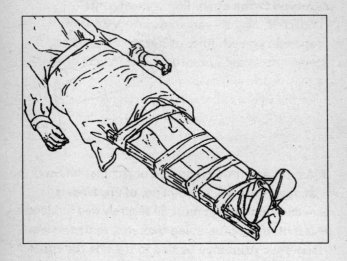

Improvised splints can be very effective in an emergency. The sound leg can also act as a splint. Good padding is important.

The principle is that to immobilize a fracture, the joint above and below the fracture must be prevented from moving.

Adequate first aid immobilization of an upper arm fracture can be achieved with two squares of cloth, each folded to form a triangular bandage.

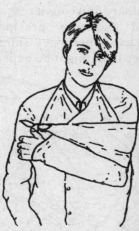

◆ Almost any firm, elongated object may be used as a splint. Plenty of padding, of any kind, is needed and splints must be securely tied in place.

◆ It is often helpful, in leg fractures, to tie the legs together. Arms may be tied to the side for upper arm fractures. A sling is usually sufficient support for a lower arm fracture.

A lower arm fracture requires only a single triangular bandage sling.

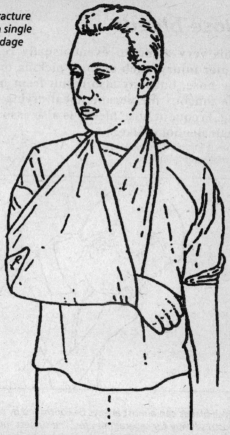

Nose bleeds

This very common event usually results from minor injury, such as nose-picking or a blow to the nose, but may also result from infection of the mucous membrane, local drying and crusting. Frequent nose bleeds is also associated with high alcohol intake.

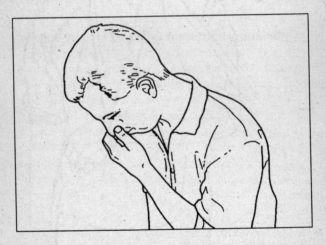

Nose bleeds can almost always be controlled by pinching the nostrils firmly for several minutes. The subject should lean forward to prevent blood running down the back of the nose.

The Priorities

Remember ABC

AIRWAY,

BREATHING and

CIRCULATION

Nose bleeding should not be considered a sign of high blood pressure although it is fairly common in people with arterial disease who may have hypertension. It can, however, be serious, and may even be life-threatening, especially in the elderly. Occasionally, nose bleed is an indication of general disease, such as atherosclerosis, a blood-clotting disorder, leukaemia or haemophilia, and it may sometimes be an indication of local disease, such as cancer (nasopharyngeal carcinoma).

◆ Nose bleeds can almost always be controlled by pinching the nostrils firmly together for five minutes and breathing through the mouth.

◆ Pressure maintained for this length of time will allow the blood to clot and the bleeding is unlikely to recur unless the site is disturbed.

◆ Failure to control bleeding by this method may call for medical attention – the bleeding area can be cauterized by touching with a tiny wool swab moistened with a corrosive chemical, or the nose may be firmly packed with ribbon gauze.

Rarely, the bleeding vessel is so far back in the nose, or so difficult to compress, that more major surgery is required. It is sometimes necessary to tie off the main artery from which the bleeding branch arises.

Bleeding in children, arising from persistent crusting of the insides of the nostrils, is best treated by the use of a softening ointment such as petroleum jelly.

Fainting

This is a temporary loss of consciousness due to a drop in the blood pressure so that the brain is deprived of an adequate supply of fuel (glucose) and oxygen. The drop in blood pressure results either from a reduction in the rate of pumping of blood by the heart or from an extensive widening of the arteries of the body.

Common faints usually occur from simultaneous slowing of the heart and widening of the arteries, often after prolonged standing, especially in hot conditions, when the return of blood to the heart by the veins is impeded.

A severe fright or shock may cause sudden slowing of the heart, by way of the nerve which controls the heart rate (the vagus nerve). Fainting is also more likely when the volume of the blood is reduced as in fluid loss from prolonged diarrhoea or excessive sweating.

Low blood pressure is normally desirable, but an abnormally low degree, as in Addison's disease or from over-enthusiastic treatment for high blood pressure, can be dangerous.

In a faint, the vision becomes misty, the ears ring, the skin becomes pale and the pulse slow. The resultant fall is exactly what is required to restore the flow of blood to the brain, and this can be encouraged by raising the legs.

Epileptic fits or convulsions are not faints and call for urgent medical attention if they do not stop within a few minutes. A prolonged series of fits is dangerous. Try to arrange the victim's surroundings so that he cannot hurt himself. Do not use a gag.

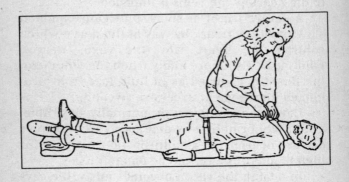

A fainting person should never be raised. Elevate the feet and loosen the clothing, then leave matters to nature.